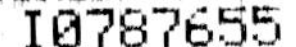

PLANT-BASED DIET SUCCESS

A FUN AND SIMPLE WAY TO LOSE WEIGHT AND FEEL GREAT FOR LIFE!

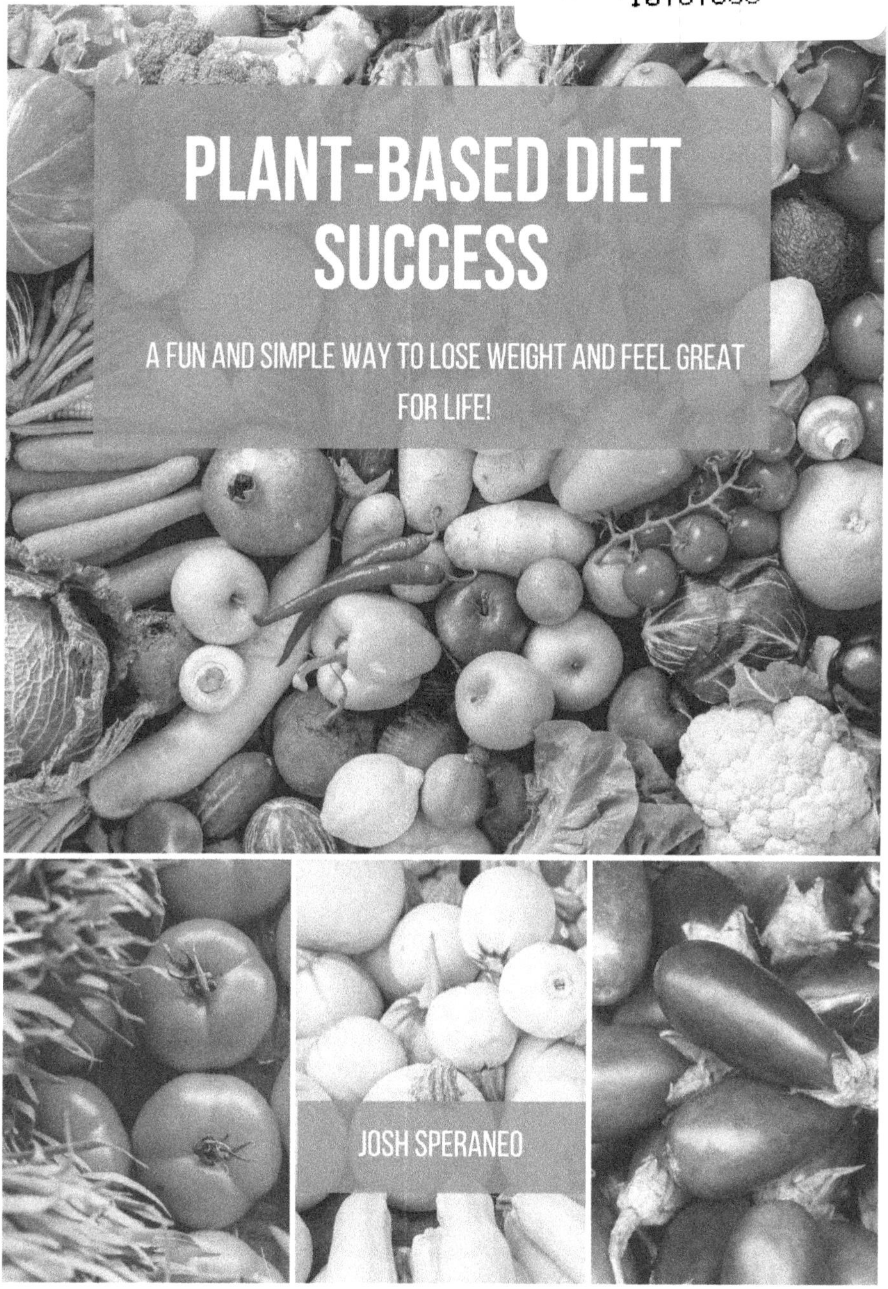

JOSH SPERANEO

<u>Plant-Based Diet Success:</u>
<u>A Fun and Simple Way to Lose Weight and Feel Great for Life!</u>

CONTENTS:

<u>**Dedication**</u>

<u>**Week 1: Mindset and Motivation**</u>

- Lesson 7: Using Grains to Fill in the Gap
    - Success Lesson 7: Visualization and Dieting

<u>Week 2: Taking Action</u>

- Lesson 8: A Little Exercise Goes A Long Way
    - Success Lesson 8: Start Small

- Lesson 9: Four Steps to Turning Your Life Around
    - Success Lesson 9: A Formula for Inspiration

- Lesson 10: One Healthy Choice After Another
    - Success Lesson 10: Your Secret Life

- Lesson 11: Discipline Makes the Difference
    - Success Lesson 11: Love and Discipline

- Lesson 12: Grocery Shopping 101
    - Success Lesson 12: Making a Meal Plan

- Lesson 13: How to Survive Eating Out
    - Success Lesson 13: Turning Mealtime into Quality Time

- Lesson 14: To Cheat or Not to Cheat?
    - Success Lesson 14: Your New Mantra

<u>Week 3: Staying Focused</u>

- Lesson 15: Halfway There!
    - Success Lesson 15: Taking Action to Achieve

DEDICATION:

To my family and friends:

Your love and encouragement inspire me to dream big dreams!

To the authors and speakers quoted in this book:

Thank you for giving me the tools to bring my dream to life!

To you:

The world is waiting for you!

You've been hiding your true self and your talents for too long.

The world needs *YOU*.

They need your words. They need your gifts.

They need your life!

For so long, you've held yourself back, afraid
of what people might say or think...

The world has been a sadder place because of it.

Step forward into your potential.

Step out into your *real* life.

Give the world the gift of your presence, your passion,
your inspiration.

And watch them come alive with joy!

Everything you've ever wanted is just ahead...

Let's go!

JOSH SPERANEO

Plant-Based Diet Success

Week 1: Mindset and Motivation

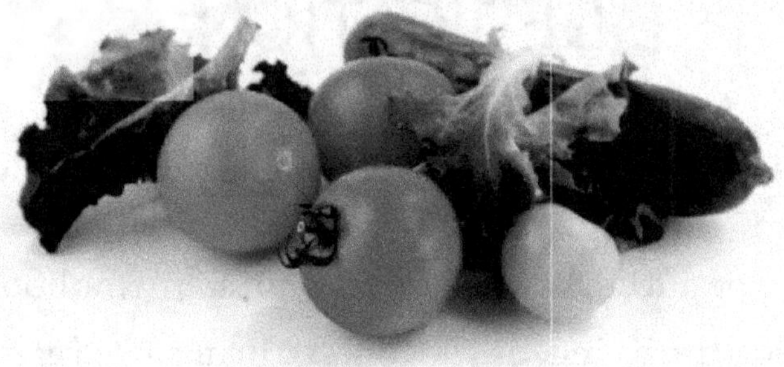

LESSON 1:

Introduction

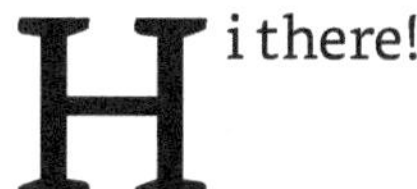 i there!

Welcome to Plant-Based Diet Success! I'm glad you're here!

In this book, you'll find the lessons I learned on my journey to weight-loss success.

Now, I have to admit that when I started out, I didn't know a whole lot about losing weight.

On an external level:

- I knew I weighed right around 244 pounds. (That might be okay for an NFL line-backer, but it's a *ton* of weight for a guy like me who's only 5 feet 6 inches tall!)
- I knew I felt tired and sluggish all the time.
- And I knew carrying around that extra weight was probably going to lead to some pretty severe health issues over time.

On an internal level:

- I knew that I had pretty much *zero* self-confidence.
- My self-image was terrible: I didn't like how I looked, or how I felt inside.

- And my self-talk was negative enough the FCC would've had to censor it if it played on the radio…

In short, I was a mess.

So, I made the decision to pursue my goal of losing weight. (I'm guessing that same decision is probably what led *you* here today).

Here's a quick riddle I heard about decisions:

Three frogs sat on a log.
One of them decided to jump off.
How many frogs are left on the log?

The answer? Still ***three***!

The point of the riddle is that one of the frogs *decided* to jump off the log, but he didn't actually *do anything*!

Where am I going with this?

Today, my scale shows that I'm weighing in right around 165 pounds.

That's right, I lost right around 33% of my total weight!

What happened? I took action!

Not only did I *decide* to lose weight, I also did whatever it took to achieve my goal of reaching my ideal weight and living a happier, healthier life. And now I'm living the life I dreamed of every single day!

This is where *you* come in!

You see, my goal was to lose weight. But my *Why* (*my core motivation*) wasn't just to get rid of the weight, it was to learn from my experience and help other people lose weight too!

That's what Plant-Based Diet Success is really about. It's all about sharing the lessons I learned along the way which helped me to lose all that weight, and *keep it off*!

- It's about helping you navigate the ups and downs of dieting.
- Helping you avoid some of the pitfalls and plateaus I ran into along the way.
- And giving you a roadmap to the life of your dreams!

That's a pretty big promise, I know. But I honestly think you'll find all of that in here—and more!

You see, what makes Plant-Based Diet Success different is the *Success* part.

Sure, I'll walk you through the steps I took to lose weight. And yes, we'll talk a little about the science behind losing weight.

But I'll also share the personal development lessons I learned along the way which helped me to transform my mental and emotional life while I was on my weight-loss journey.

I believe these lessons can make all the difference when it comes to not only *losing* the weight, but also *keeping it off*.

Sound like a plan?

Ready to get started?

Great!

Let's dive in!

To **your** success!

Josh

SUCCESS LESSON 1:

A 30-Day Challenge

I want to begin by giving you the same challenge I gave myself when I started my plant-based diet.

Here it is: For the next 30 days, I challenge you to cut out all meat and dairy products from your meals. I also challenge you to cut out sugary soft drinks and fattening desserts.

Instead, only eat foods that fall into one of these categories: fruits, vegetables, grains, nuts, and legumes. And only drink water or fruit juice. (If you're a caffeine addict, pick up a drink mix you can add into your water that has caffeine in it).

This is how I launched my diet, and it made a huge difference in my success. I told myself, "I'll try a plant-based diet for 30 days and see how it goes. If it's working, I'll stick with it. If not, at least I can say I tried."

I ended up losing 14 pounds in 14 days!

Not a bad start, right?

Now, I can't guarantee those results for everyone. However, I honestly believe that this diet will work for anyone who gives it an honest chance.

And, in reality, you're not just giving the *diet* a chance, you're giving *yourself* a chance.

- A chance to prove you can lose those unwanted pounds.
- A chance to prove you can achieve your weight-loss goal.
- A chance to prove you're serious about wanting to live a happier, healthier life.

Don't worry, you're not going to be alone on this journey. I'll be here with you every step of the way!

In fact, I'll be here every morning, waiting to give you the advice and insights I gained on my own journey. That way your path to diet success can be even straighter than mine was.

So, are you up to the challenge?

If so, let's spend a little time on your inner game, and then we'll dive into some tips on how you can change your eating habits, your thinking habits, and (ultimately) your life!

Now, for those of you who might be freaking out, just breathe...

If 30 days seems like a lot to ask, trust me, I understand.

I have no doubt that committing to only eating a plant-based diet for 30 straight days helped to launch me on my way to diet success.

However, I realize not everybody's ready to completely over-haul their eating choices in one day.

Why don't we compromise?

If you're not feeling up to the 30- Day Challenge, but you still want to give a plant-based diet a try, start small.

Try replacing a few meals a week with plant-based alternatives and see how you feel.

If you find yourself feeling better, replace a few more meals each week.

You might want to start with your morning meals, or you may

have more luck adjusting your mid-day meals. It's much easier to stay consistent when you're eating at home, so that's usually the best place to start. If you cut yourself some slack when you're out and about, I certainly won't judge you.

The important thing is to give your plant-based diet a fair chance. From there, the results you'll see will speak for themselves and springboard you on your way to diet success!

LESSON 2:

The Catalyst

It seems like everyone I've talked to who's tried to lose weight has a story of an experience that pushed them across the line from thinking about losing weight, to deciding they had to do something about their weight.

What's *your* story?

What was the moment that made you think, "I *have* to get this weight off?"

- Maybe it was your doctor's advice.
- Maybe it was something a friend or family member (or even a stranger) said.
- Or maybe it was an embarrassing situation in public—like not being able to ride a ride at an amusement park because the restraint wouldn't fit.

Before you start to think that I'm somehow different or special, let me share my catalyst with you:

I have a friend with seven kids that vary in age from 6 to 18. (Crazy, right?)

Anyway, here's what happened: One day, when I was over at their house, the enormity of my excess weight hit me.

You see, as I was playing with his kids (including giving the inevitable piggy-back rides), I realized that it was basically like I was walking around with his eight-year-old son on my shoulders *all the time!*

Have you had a moment like this?

A moment where you picked up something heavy and thought, *"Wow, I'm carrying around this much extra weight all the time!"*

Think about it:

- Maybe it's a case of bottled water.
- Maybe it's a bag of cat food.
- Maybe it's something heavier like your own child, or a niece or nephew.

The point is, carrying around all that extra weight is *exhausting!*

The good news is that walking around without that extra weight is *liberating!*

Not sure where to start?

That's where I come in.

Throughout this book, I'll share with you how I was able to shed more than 70 pounds over the course of 18 months, and how I've kept the weight off.

And, while I can't guarantee you'll see the same results, I can tell you with certainty that if you keep doing what you've been doing, you'll keep getting what you've always gotten (or worse).

This leads us to…

SUCCESS LESSON 2:

Start by Taking Full Responsibility

For those of you who've read Jack Canfield's book The Success Principles: How to Get from Where You Are to Where You Want to Be, you'll realize that this idea is at the core of success.

It seems like a great place for *us* to start too!

You see, as long as we're looking for someone else to blame for where we are in life, or we're making excuses about why we *can't* change, we won't be able to make progress toward our weight-loss goals.

So, starting today, let's own where we are in terms of our weight. Maybe that's 10 pounds heavier than you want to be, or maybe you feel like you're closer to 50 pounds over your ideal weight.

Those numbers aren't nearly as important as this realization: *If I'm responsible for the decisions that led me to my current weight, then I can make better decisions that will lead me to my ideal weight.*

Let that sink in, because as soon as you take responsibility for where you are, you can begin making the changes that will get you where you want to be!

If you're ready to start making these changes, come with me, and I'll tell you about the changes I made (inside and out) that

JOSH SPERANEO

changed my life.

LESSON 3:

"I Can't Get There from Here..."

Have you had this thought when it comes to weight-loss?

I know I did.

I'd think about how heavy I was and what my ideal weight was, and it seemed like there was a huge chasm I couldn't cross...

Which leads me to one of the truths about successful weight-loss: It's **never** an overnight thing. It takes time and consistent good choices to get there.

Here's another truth (from this side of weight-loss): It's totally worth the effort to reach your goal and live a happier, healthier life!

For so many of us, we picture the future we want, and we see ourselves being physically fit and healthy. Then we look at reality and think, "There's no way I'll ever get there..."

But there *is* a way!

No, I don't have a magic pill to offer you. I'm also not aware of an Easy Button you can push to get to your ideal weight.

Here's what I *can* offer you:

- I can give you the plan I used to lose over 70 pounds (and keep it off afterward).

- I can give you support and encouragement.
- And I can give you the lessons I learned along my weight-loss journey.

Think of this as a crossroads:

Option One: You can keep going down the road you've been on. (But you know where that road goes, don't you? More of the same…)

Option Two: You can pull over and wait for them to discover some new medical technique where they'll put you to sleep and you'll wake up at your ideal weight.

Or, Option Three: Start down this road with me. Keep your 30-day challenge going and see if you start to feel better and make progress toward your weight-loss goals.

You can always come back to this intersection and take a different path, but if you turn away now, you'll never know if this could have been the way to the future you've dreamed of.

So, what do you say? Are you ready to cross that chasm?

SUCCESS LESSON 3:

Your Ideal Weight

Before we go on to our next lesson, take a second to think about where you want to end up: Your ideal weight.

Do you have a number in mind? A goal you're shooting for?

Only you can know what your ideal weight really is. And, in truth, you may not even know until you get there.

My advice is this: rather than look at the BMI (which I'm not a fan of), think about the time in your life when you felt the most physically fit:

- Maybe it was in high school.
- Maybe it was in your 20's.
- Or maybe it was even a little later than that.

How would you like to get back to *that* weight?

I know it may sound too good to be true, but stick with me here!

You see, this is exactly what I was able to do by following a plant-based diet.

Without even realizing it, I lost weight until I went right past what I believed my ideal weight was, and ended up back at (or a little below) my weight when I was playing tennis in high school!

So, don't be afraid to think big here! As Norman Vincent Peale said, "Shoot for the moon. Even if you miss, you'll land among the stars."

Whatever number you come up with, hold onto it. We'll refer back to it soon!

LESSON 4:

Find Your Reason Why

Today, I want to offer you an insight you won't find with most other diet plans. You see, those plans will offer you the usual advice:

- Eat this.
- Don't eat *that*.
- And we'll cover those things soon…

But what most of those plans **won't** cover is the importance of finding *your reason Why*.

Success coach Jim Rohn said, "Reasons come first, answers come second."

Your Why is what will get you through the hard times.

It's the thing that will keep you going when the going gets tough.

It's like a compass that keeps you moving in the right direction when distractions and temptations come. *And they will*!

As John Assaraf likes to say, "Your motivation is *your motive for action*!"

Here are some powerful ways to help you get started thinking about your own Why:

It could be External:

- To be able to play with your kids (or grandkids) without getting winded.
- To lose enough weight to get the knee surgery you need.
- To fit into those clothes in your closet that hang there and haunt you because you either used to fit into them or you wish you could.
- To be able to ride that new ride at the amusement park!

Or it could be <u>Internal</u>:

- To feel confident about your body again.
- To know that you look great in your favorite outfit!
- To have more energy.
- To stop feeling so self-conscious all the time.
- To find a new sense of life and passion!
- To prove to yourself (*and others*) you can do it!

Now, think about your own Why.

Fill in this blank: I want to lose weight so I can ___________________. That's your Why!

It's the reason that will keep you going when you feel like giving up!

Think of it as your North Star. Let it give you a sense of direction and motivation so you can stay on course toward your goal.

Take your time while you think about your Why.

Don't rush this part of your journey.

Too many people start a diet program without taking this step, and then give up because they lose sight of their reason for staying the course.

Don't let that be *your* story.

Instead, decide today why you want to lose the weight. Make sure it's something *powerful and meaningful*. Think about what a happier healthier life looks like for you.

Go ahead, dream a little!

- What are you doing?
- Where are you going?
- Who are you with?

That's *your* Why.

Now, let's get you there!

SUCCESS LESSON 4:

Your Weight-Loss Affirmation

Writing an affirmation is as simple as stating your goal as though you've already achieved it. However, the power of affirmations goes far beyond this.

You see, when you set a goal, your brain immediately looks at that goal and decides whether or not to accept it. (For incredible information about how our brain processes goals, check out John Assaraf's book <u>Innercise: The New Science to Unlock Your Brain's Hidden Power</u>).

For many of us, setting a weight-loss goal triggers the fear center in our brain.

We say, "I want to weigh 180 pounds!" And our brain says, "Nope. Can't do it. You can't get *there* from *here*."

But, if we send the same message to our brain as an affirmation, not only can we get our brain on board with the goal, it will actually look for ways to help us get there!

It's pretty incredible stuff when your inner critic suddenly becomes your inner coach!

Here's how you put together your personal weight-loss affirmation:

First, think back to the ideal weight you wrote down before.

Second, add your Why.

Now, frame it up like this:

"I'm so happy and grateful that I've reached my ideal weight of <u>X</u> pounds, and now I'm enjoying <u>(insert your why)</u>!"

For example: "I'm so happy and grateful that I've reached my ideal weight of 165 pounds, and now I'm filled with the self-confidence to pursue all my goals and dreams!"

Or: "I'm so happy and grateful that I've reached my ideal weight of 175 pounds, and now I'm enjoying flying a kite in the park with my grandkids!"

What is your affirmation? Be sure to write it down and share it with someone you trust. (Sharing goals increases the likelihood we'll follow through in achieving them).

Now, here's where the real power comes in. After you write out your affirmation, commit to reading it out loud two or three times a day.

- Carry it with you in your wallet or phone case.
- Set it as your screen saver.
- Put a note on your bathroom mirror.
- Whatever works best for you.

The important thing is to *keep it where you'll see it*!

Then, when you read it out, trace over it with your finger to imprint it more deeply into your brain.

Lastly, and possibly *most importantly*, take a few moments to visualize what it will look like to achieve your goal and let yourself *feel the feelings* you'll feel when you've achieved your Why!

Does this sound a little crazy? Trust me, it's not. This method is actually backed by neuroscience.

Plus, what do you have to lose?

For now, just promise me you'll give it a try and see what happens.

And don't forget to share your Why, so your friends and family can support you as you work toward making your weight-loss goals a reality!

LESSON 5:

The Power of Consistency

Now that you have a picture of the future you want, let's work on getting you there!

How are we going to do that?

Small disciplines practiced consistently one day at a time.

What are these disciplines?

They're healthy choices you make from moment to moment that lead from where you are to where you want to be.

1. <u>Drink as few empty calories as possible</u> - This means that sugary sodas have to go.

   When you drink a can of Coke, you're adding 140 empty calories to your meal. You're also drinking 8 teaspoons of sugar.

What if you're out to eat and you get a refill? That's 280 extra calories and 16 teaspoons of sugar. It adds up fast!

Think of it this way: one sugar cube is 1 teaspoon of sugar. So, every time you drink a soda, it's like sucking down 8 sugar cubes. *Yuck!*

2. <u>Start walking</u> - How much? As much as you can.

If you can walk 5 miles a day, that's great! If you can only walk half a mile a day, that's okay too.

Physical activity is extremely important when it comes to losing weight.

Will you see results if all you do is change your diet? It's entirely possible, but walking (or working in some other exercise) can *dramatically improve* your results!

If walking is too hard on your knees, consider buying a recumbent exercise bike or swimming, or finding some other way to get moving and burn off calories.

Our goal is to fight calories on both fronts: Eating and drinking less and burning off more.

3. <u>Say goodbye to meat and dairy products</u>- This one factor will dramatically reduce the number of calories, carbs, and fats you take in on a daily basis.

    Is it a major life change for many people? Yes.

    Was it hard for me? Absolutely!

    Do I regret letting go of meat and dairy products and losing over 70 pounds? Not at all.

    And neither will you when you reach your weight-loss goal!

Plus, in addition to weight-loss, studies have shown that cutting out meat and dairy products can also help in these areas:

- Lowering cholesterol
- Lowering your risk of heart disease
- Lowering high blood-pressure
- Lowering your risk of getting certain cancers
- Lowering your risk of developing diabetes (or

    lowering the severity of symptoms for those
with diabetes)

- Decreasing chronic pain for people who struggle with arthritis, migraines, or conditions caused by inflammation in their joints
- It may even reduce your risk of developing Alzheimer's disease!

(You can find more information on the studies behind these statements in books like <u>The Vegan Starter Kit </u> by Neal D. Barnard, MD or <u>The Healthspan Solution</u> by Julieanna Hever and Ray Cronise).

4. <u>Make room for fruits, veggies, legumes, and grains!</u>

> As a part of this process, you need to purge your cabinets of anything that doesn't fit into your diet. You can give them away to friends and family or donate them somewhere, but they need to go. Otherwise, the temptation to go back to unhealthy eating may be too strong.

> What if you live with people who aren't going on this diet with you?

> You'll have to be very focused and disciplined to keep from going back to old habits. You may even have to start labeling your food and keeping it separate.

A friend of mine doing this diet would fix dinner for her kids and then make her own meal afterward. It was a challenge at first, but eventually they found a new rhythm.
If you're still in shock about giving up meat and dairy products, take a deep breath. We'll go over some action steps to help make your transition to plant-based foods easier in just a little while.

*Hopefully the name of the book gave you a clue that this was going to happen... :)

OK, so we've ditched the sugary soft drinks. We've gotten more physically active. And we've given away our meat and dairy products.

Is that it? No.

5. <u>Send out the sweets</u> - Now it's time to toss the Twinkies, cast out the cookies, and incinerate the ice cream. (Sorry, I needed an *I* word).
    The moral of the story is to get rid of any sugary/fattening desserts.

    This also includes snack cakes. Those little guys pack a lot of empty calories, and they can throw your diet off-track very quickly.

6. <u>Alcohol may be your enemy</u> - Many beers contain just as many calories as soft drinks (or more).

    Drinking these extra calories is like trying to run a race with a backpack full of bricks. It'll hold you back the whole time you're trying to move forward.

Now, keep in mind, I'm not going to come to your house and go through your cabinets. So, I'll never know whether or not you actually went through this purging process.

But remember two things:
- First, you purchased this book because you want a better life, and that means giving up eating and drinking for entertainment and focusing on making better nutritional choices instead.
- Second, you have to keep your eye on your Why at times like this.

    Is it hard? Heck yeah!

    Why do you think so many people give up on diets and walk around overweight or obese?

But that's not how *your* story goes!

You've looked ahead.

You know where you're headed.

And this is the first major step on your journey to your ideal weight!

Clearing out your cabinets to make room for healthy foods allows you to open the doors to a whole new life! A life of consistent, healthy choices that lead to the future you've dreamed of.

Don't cheat yourself by making excuses here and holding onto unhealthy foods and habits. Let them go, so you can move forward into your new life!

SUCCESS LESSON 5:

*Making the Switch to Healthier
Eating Habits*

When it comes to changing your habits, few people have done more research than James Clear. He's the author of Atomic Habits: Tiny Changes, Remarkable Results. (I highly recommend that you pick up a copy or listen to the audiobook!)

In his book, Clear highlights the keys to breaking bad habits and instilling good ones with incredible insight and clarity.

For our purposes, I'll just highlight a few thoughts from the book:

- Our habits go through a predictable 4-stage cycle (The Habit Loop): Cue, Craving, Response, Reward.

- If we want to get rid of a bad habit, we can weaken it at any of those four stages:
  1. Cue- Make it invisible
  2. Craving- Make it unattractive
  3. Response- Make it difficult
  4. Reward- Make it unsatisfying

- In the same way, if we want to reinforce a good habit, we can strengthen it at any of those four stages:

1. Cue- Make it obvious
2. Craving- Make it attractive
3. Response- Make it easy
4. Reward- Make it satisfying

So, when we're working on developing healthier eating habits, we can use Clear's Habit Loop to our advantage.

- Take control of your Cues- Do your best to remove any foods that aren't plant-based from your home (make them invisible). (Or, like we talked about, at least remove them from *your* section of the fridge or pantry). Then replace them with healthy substitutes. For example, you could put a bowl of your favorite fruit on your kitchen table (make it obvious).

- Expect to experience Cravings- Like it or not, cravings are going to happen. One way to fight them is to keep an unflattering picture of you at your starting weight close by and look at it when you're tempted to eat something off-diet (make it unattractive). Then, when you choose to eat something healthy instead, look at a picture that reminds you of your Why (make it attractive).

- Be careful to plan your Responses- How difficult is it for you to access junk food? For most people, it's as simple as a quick walk to the kitchen. That's why getting rid of unhealthy food choices is so essential. If you can't remove them from your home completely (i.e. because the people you live with might *riot*), then at least make it more of a challenge to get to it.
"But what about when people bring donuts to the office, or I'm eating out?" you might ask. I'll give you some tips and strategies for those types of scenarios later.

- Focus on positive Rewards- Every habit has a reward. And, more often than not, our habits revolve around some kind of instant gratification. As Clear says, "The consequences of bad habits are delayed, while the rewards are immediate."
Herein lies our struggle: the battle between Future You and Present You.

But how do we win this battle? Clear says our best bet is to, "Add a little bit of immediate pleasure to the habits that pay off in the long run, and a little bit of immediate pain to the ones that don't."

The key is a feeling of success! "Immediate reinforcement helps maintain motivation in the short-term, while you're waiting for the long-term rewards to arrive." This immediate reinforcement can take many forms.

Here are some suggestions, based on recommendations from Atomic Habits, but applied to our goal of losing weight:

A. Create a "New Wardrobe Jar." Then, whenever you pass up on eating ice cream or cake, put $5 in the jar. That way you're rewarding yourself for your good choices, and saving up for clothes that you'll love once you've reached your ideal weight.

Trust me, when I went from XL shirts and 36-30 pants to medium shirts and 32-30 pants, I wished I had saved up!

B. When your family's bringing out the ice cream after dinner, use that time to go for a quiet walk or sneak away to take a peaceful bubble bath.

C. Do something else that makes you feel good. For example, if you love encouraging people, you could keep a stack of cards where you used to keep your sweets. Then, when you open up that cabinet, instead of grabbing a snack cake, you can write an encouraging card or thank-you note to a friend or co-worker. If you love music, take some time to download some new songs from your favorite artists. If you're like me, and you love reading, go browse on Amazon and add a few more books to your wish list.

In the end, keep in mind that our bad habits didn't form overnight, so we probably won't overcome them in a single day. But, by following the strategies outlined in <u>Atomic Habits</u>, we can at least give ourselves a fighting chance of trading the habits that are holding us back for more empowering habits that will help us reach our weight-loss goals.

LESSON 6:

The Importance of Planning

Now that you've gotten rid of the food and drinks that were holding you back, it's time to restock your pantry and fridge with groceries that will help you reach your goals.

Here are some guidelines to help you get started:

1. <u>Water, water everywhere!</u> Drink as much water as you can.

"But what if I don't like drinking water?" you might ask.

I don't either, but there are all sorts of zero calorie drink enhancers you can put into your water to give it flavor. As I mentioned before, some of these mixes also contain caffeine, which is helpful for those of us who are used to drinking soda to get our caffeine fix.

2. <u>Bring in the fruits</u>- Fresh fruit is great to have on hand for snacks and sides or as a substitute for sugary desserts. You can also keep canned fruit on hand and put together a fruit salad when you're fighting a craving or trying to satisfy your sweet tooth.

3. <u>Get all of the vegetables you can stand</u>- I realize this

will be a challenge for many people. Most of us have a few different veggies where we draw the line.

Your nemesis may be peas or Brussels sprouts or lima beans or broccoli. And that's fine.

Just stock up on all of the others (especially salads and leafy greens). You can eat a lot of these foods and still take in a minimal amount of calories—which is exactly what we're looking for!

4. <u>Grains are good too</u>- We don't want to overdo it in this area, but good/whole grains will go a long way in helping you reach your weight-loss goals.

   Use them to balance out your meals and help make sure you're not starving yourself.

5. <u>Satisfying snacks</u>- Nuts and veggie-based chips or crackers are great to have on hand when cravings strike. Just be sure you know what your portion sizes are for these, so you don't go overboard.

6. <u>Dressings, dips, spreads, and spices</u>– "Everything in moderation" is important here.

   First, you want to make sure they qualify as plant-based. Then, you want to keep an eye on the calories.

   A healthy salad can quickly get overloaded with the wrong dressing. And a dip or sauce can add too many calories and hold you back from making progress toward your goals.

   Don't let the desire to entertain your taste buds trip you up!

I realize a lot of the changes I'm suggesting are drastic.

Remember, I've been where you are. I understand that giving up certain foods and drinks can be extremely challenging.

We're naturally creatures of habit, so we tend to eat the same things week after week; at home, as well as when we're eating out.

That's why I recommend purging your kitchen of all the unhealthy food and drinks you've been consuming.

If it's not there, you can't eat or drink it.

- Want a snack cake? Too bad, they're gone.
- Want a soda? Oh, those are gone too.
- Want a burger or some chicken strips? Can't help you there, sorry.
- Cookies and milk? We're all out.

Getting rid of those things will save you thousands of potential empty calories every week.

Where you used to have a 900 to 1500 calorie breakfast, you'll have a 300 to 500 calorie breakfast instead.

"What if I'm still hungry?"

If you surround yourself with low calorie foods and snacks, then you can eat a little more and still be just fine.

*Here's a challenge I used to give myself: Try to eat the same kind of portions today that you'll be eating when you reach your ideal weight.

Does that sound impossible? It's really not.

And, each time you do it, you're not only increasing your willpower, you're also giving yourself a huge boost toward your goal.

You'll notice that in situations where you used to eat everything on your plate, you'll start eating less of your food and taking home leftovers instead.

Or (and this will come as a shock to some) *just let it go*. Leave it behind or throw it away.

Making good choices about what *not* to eat can help as well.

It's strangely empowering to think, "I used to eat that whole steak an both sides, but today I only ordered the two sides and I feel great!"

That's the power you'll find when you begin controlling your portions and planning for your success.

SUCCESS LESSON 6:

Start at the End of the Story

One of the easiest ways to make good choices is by beginning with the end in mind.

Those of you who've read Stephen R. Covey's <u>The 7 Habits of Highly Effective People</u> will recognize this thought as the second habit from that book.

I wanted to include this lesson here in order to make a connection between the dietary changes I'm asking you to make and the vision for the future I asked you to come up with earlier: Your Why.

As Covey says, "It means to know where you're going so that you better understand where you are now and so that the steps you take are always in the right direction."

Think about it, how many people set a new year's resolution to lose weight, only to give up within a few days, or (at best) a few weeks into the new year?

That's where beginning with the end in mind comes in.

I'll repeat this point a few times throughout this book: Having a clear vision of where you're going helps you say No to bad dietary decisions because you've already said Yes to your goal.

Envisioning the future of your dreams puts everything in perspective. In every situation you can ask, "Does this move me closer to my goal of losing weight, or will it hold me back?"

That's why it's so essential to keep your affirmation where you can see it, and to stay laser-focused on your Why.

Let's be realistic. Challenges *will* come up along the way.

- You'll end up at your favorite restaurant.
- Your mom will offer to cook your favorite meal.
- Your favorite dessert will get served at Thanksgiving dinner.
- Your coworkers will bring in donuts, or cookies, or cake (oh my!)

The easiest way to turn these things down in those moments of temptation is by focusing on where you want to end up.

So, say No, because you've already said Yes!

LESSON 7:

Using Grains to Fill in the Gap

Many people will consider starting on a plant-based diet, but then give it up because they "can't survive on rabbit food!" But a plant-based diet consists of a huge variety of foods.

For instance, many of my favorite plant-based meals involve wheat or rice.

Our goal is to avoid meat and dairy products and sweets.

That leaves grains, beans, rice, and nuts all on the table (in reasonable portions).

- Whole grain crackers are fine.
- Pinto beans and rice are good.
- Potatoes and sweet potatoes are okay.
- And, unless you're allergic, nuts can be your new best friend.

Don't focus on the *cant's*, focus on the *cans*. And make sure you stop to check the label on a product if you're not sure if it fits your diet.

Don't just assume that because you enjoyed something before your diet that you "probably can't have it now." This kind of mindset focuses on what you're giving up and makes you more susceptible to cheating or quitting.

Keep your eyes on your end goal and explore the full range of foods you can enjoy on your way there.

You might just pick up some new favorites that'll stick with you even after you reach your weight-loss goals. I know I have!

In the end, I hope you'll find (as I did) that there is a nearly endless list of potential foods you can incorporate into your meal plan. And there is always a new twist to add to your favorite dishes.

Don't be afraid to try new things either! You may discover that you really like quinoa or that broccoli isn't as bad as you thought it was.

Finding new variations on lettuce wraps, making plant-based sandwiches on wheat bread, or using whole wheat tortillas can provide you with a huge variety of options.

There's also a wide range of plant-based diet friendly spreads and dressings to add flavor to your favorite dishes.

Keep an open mind and try new things. When you find a solid list of favorites, start rotating them from day to day and week to week so you don't burn out.

*Just remember, our goal is low calories and reasonable portions. We're eating to fuel our bodies and keep going towards our goal. We're *not* eating for entertainment.

Even so, have fun with this! There are a lot more plant-based options out there than you might think!

SUCCESS LESSON 7:

Visualization and Dieting

"**O**h, now you're going to get all new-agey on me!" you might be thinking. That's not my intent, but I believe there's power in casting a vision and picturing where you want to go.

Think about your diet journey as a road trip. You can take all sorts of routes to get where you want to go.

However, my hope is that this book will serve as a kind of GPS system to help you avoid some of the wrong turns and dead ends I (and others like me) have run into along the way.

Visualization is key because it's a way for us to picture ourselves in the future.

Think about it for a second: What will your life look like 5 years from now?

- Still overweight?
- Clothes still too tight?
- Squeezing into booths at restaurants?
- Uncomfortable with your size?

Or maybe you've reached your ideal weight.

- You are healthy and happy.
- You have all kinds of energy and there's a big smile on

your face!

- You are more agile and attractive than you've been in years.

All of this shows in how you carry yourself and how you treat the people around you. You've learned to love yourself again (inside and out) and everyone can see it!

In visualizing the future you want, you're training your subconscious to head in that direction. You're telling yourself, "That's where I want to go!" And your mind will do everything it can to help you reach that goal.

It may sound strange, but don't underestimate the power of this discipline. Give it a try. Each night before you go to bed, take a few minutes to visualize what you want your life to be like five years from now.

Think about your weight, but also think about the overall life you want to be experiencing as well.

Play yourself a mental movie of your perfect day in your ideal future.

- What's life like from the time you wake up until the time you go back to bed?
- How is that day different from your life today?
- What changes do you need to make to reach the life of your dreams?

Think back to the earlier lesson where we talked about finding your Why.

Now use your Why to paint a picture of the future of your dreams.

You wouldn't have set a goal there that you didn't think you could achieve, so now is the time to get a really vivid mental picture of your Why and keep it in front of you to keep you moving forward.

You may even want to find a picture in a magazine that represents where you're hoping to go and put it up somewhere to remind you every day what you're working toward.

For example: If your Why involves spending more time playing with your children or grandchildren, make sure you keep a picture of them nearby all the time so you can look at it and remind yourself why it's important to stick with your goals.

*If you can find a picture that triggers positive emotions like joy or excitement, *that's even better!*

And remember, the most important piece is to picture yourself *having already achieved your goal* and enjoying the life of your dreams today.

This vision of your future will help guide your dietary decisions and keep you going through the ups and downs of weigh-ins and the sudden cravings that are sure to come.

Plant-Based Diet Success

Week 2: Taking Action

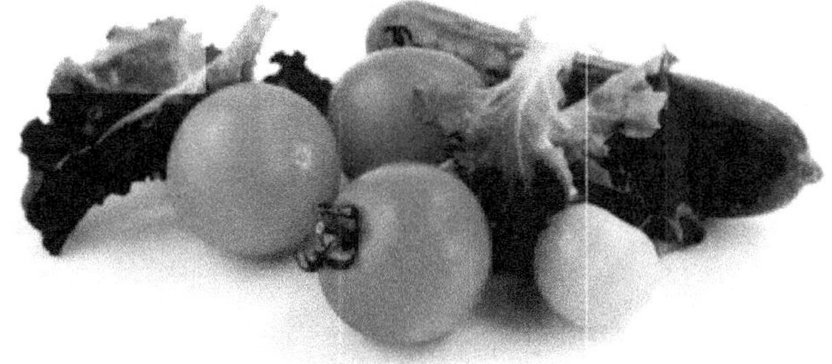

LESSON 8:

A Little Exercise Goes A Long Way

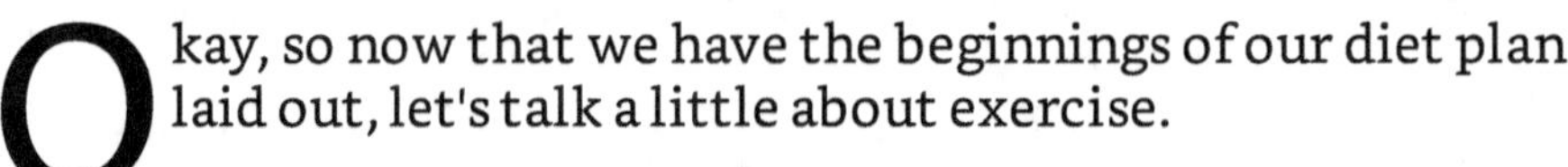

Okay, so now that we have the beginnings of our diet plan laid out, let's talk a little about exercise.

Now, I realize not everyone's ready to hop up after this lesson and go run a few miles.

Don't worry, I won't ask you to do that.

All I'm asking you to do is *as much as you feel like you can.*

If that starts with parking a little further from the store or taking the stairs instead of the elevator, that's fine.

*You know what an exercise victory would look like for you, so aim for that.

Here's the deal when it comes to exercise: *anything* is better than doing nothing.

Whether it's walking, jogging, running, biking, stair-climbing, square dancing, skating, swimming, weightlifting, or jump-roping - anything you can do to burn a few extra calories helps!

Think of this as a way to really hit the accelerator on your journey to your ideal weight!

Now, with that being said, can you still get there even if you're limited on the exercise you can do?

Sure! It may just take a little longer.

Start small and work your way up.

I once heard a man share the story of how he started running. His first day, he went outside and jogged a lap around his block. (It was actually more walking than jogging, but it was still a victory, because he did *something*!) Eventually, he worked his way up to two laps, then three, and so on. When he told this story to the group I was in, he was jogging a couple miles a day - and he was in his late 60's. He started small and raised the bar slightly until he reached his goal—and you can do the same thing!

Today, I'd like you to decide what your exercise of choice will be.

Walking has worked great for me, but you can choose whatever you'd like.

Then think about a goal you'd like to reach with your exercise. It could be swimming 10 laps or jogging two miles without stopping to walk.

Remember, it's *your* goal.

Now, what's the smallest increment you can break that goal down to?

- Swimming the length of the pool one way?
- Walking a lap around your block?

Anything's a victory if it's more than you've been doing up to this point.

Once you're hitting that goal consistently, the challenge is to take it up a notch at a time on your way to your ideal weight.

SUCCESS LESSON 8:

Start Small

In his book Tiny Habits: The Small Changes That Change Everything, B.J. Fogg explains how making small changes can bring about major results in your life.

Here's an example. Let's say you want to start exercising, but you're having trouble getting motivated.

Instead of setting the goal of jogging two miles, just focus on putting on your running shoes and tying the laces.

That's it.

No, *really*, that's it.

Here's another example. Let's say your dentist has told you that you *have* to start flossing your teeth every day. Fogg would say that you should set the goal of flossing one tooth.

Yep. One tooth.

Now, here's why this technique is powerful: What are the odds that you'll put on your running shoes and stop there?

Or how likely is it that you'll floss *one* tooth and then throw the floss in the trash?

The truth is, sometimes just getting started working on a habit is enough to launch us into practicing it regularly.

Let's look at this from an exercising perspective:

Some people will go through this lesson and then go out and jog a couple miles

Other people are getting exhausted just from seeing the word "exercise" so many times in one sitting.

If you fall into this second category, here's my challenge to you: *start one tiny habit today.*

- It could be to go put on your running shoes.
- It could be to do two push-ups as soon as you get out of bed.
- It could be to go outside and pick up three sticks or walnuts out of your yard.

As John Assaraf says, "Consistency is more important than intensity!"

Pick one activity. Start super-small. Do it consistently.

And, for accountability purposes, be sure to let other people know what activity you're committing to. Writing down your goal and sharing it with someone else are great ways to increase the likelihood that you'll follow through on it!

LESSON 9:

*Four Steps to Turning
Your Life Around*

One of Jim Rohn's most popular teachings was entitled, "The Day That Turns Your Life Around."

In this lesson, I'd like to apply the principles he shared in that talk to our diet journey.

1. <u>Disgust</u>- It starts with getting disgusted with where we're at in life. This disgust might be triggered by the number on the scale, the looks from people passing by, the button that pops off of another pair of pants, or seeing how big we've gotten when our family pictures come back.

   Whatever this trigger event might be, it leaves us saying, "Enough is enough! I have to do something about this!"

That leads us to Step 2.

2. <u>Decision</u>- It's one thing to realize that we need to change. It's a completely different thing to *make the decision* to start changing our behaviors and living differently.

Lots of people "want to lose weight." They know they need to change how they're living, but they never *actually* take any actions to shed their extra pounds.

*That's like acknowledging that the building you're in is on fire, but continuing to sit there until you burn up.

We have to decide that we want a better life for ourselves and then do what it takes to get it!

3. <u>Desire</u>- What do you desire?

    What's your Why?

    Your reason for losing the weight? The thing that fuels your passion to improve yourself and make the changes necessary to achieve the life you've always dreamed of?

    A strong desire can carry you through the ups and downs of dieting until you reach the goal you've been pursuing.

4. <u>Resolve</u>- "Resolve is promising yourself you'll never give up," as Jim Rohn quotes in his teaching.

    Have you made that promise to yourself? Have you set your heart on achieving your weight-loss goals *no matter what*?

    There will always be reasons to stop.

    "It's too hard!"
    "I'm too tired."
    "I just can't lose weight like everyone else!"

Those excuses are almost always nonsense!

You *can* do this!
You have what it takes!

> And you're just as capable of reaching your goals as anyone else!

As Jim said, the key to a good resolution is the word "Until".

"I'll keep eating healthy foods *until* the weight comes off."

"I'll keep fighting the urge to give up *until* I reach my ideal weight!"

This kind of resolve is what separates successful dieters from the unsuccessful.

It's what helps you pick yourself back up after failures.

It's what keeps you going through the sweat and tears.

And it all starts on The Day That Turns Your Life Around.

SUCCESS LESSON 9:

A Formula for Inspiration

One of the best success lessons I've come across lately is from a book called <u>The Disney Way: Harnessing The Management Secrets Of Disney In Your Company</u> by Bill Capodagli and Lynn Jackson.

Early in their book, they share a quote that's attributed to Walt Disney which speaks to the secret of his success. Disney said, "I dream, I test my dreams against my beliefs, I dare to take risks, and I execute my vision to make those dreams come true."

Or, in essence: *"Dream, Believe, Dare, Do."*

When it comes to losing weight (or any other dream we might have), it's so easy to lose momentum.

- Maybe we share our vision with someone, and they tell us it'll never happen.
- Maybe we face a setback, and our self-confidence wavers.
- Maybe the changes we need to make seem too risky, so we step back into our comfort zone.
- Or maybe we don't see the progress we're hoping for, so we give up on our dream (and ourselves).

If you're like me, you've probably run into one (or all) of these obstacles in the past. You had a dream or a goal that you believed in so strongly that you knew you *had* to take action, but then somehow life came along and knocked that dream right out of you...

Not this time!

Remember, this is the day that turns your life around! This is the day that everything changes for you!

This is *your dream*, and you're not going to stop until you bring it to life and show the world that you can accomplish *anything* you set your mind to!

So, let's take another look at Walt's formula for success:

Dream- Keep your vision of the future (your Why) in the front of your mind.

Believe- Read your affirmation *every day* and believe that you can and *will* accomplish it!

Dare- Fix your eyes on your goal and decide that *nothing's* going to stop you from reaching it.

Do- Commit to taking action every day, so you can live the life you've dreamed of.

Remember, in the same way that a seed planted in the ground takes time to break the surface and show signs of growth, you may not see the kind of progress you're hoping for after a single week.

It may take two weeks, or a month, before you really start to build momentum. However, once that momentum starts to build, you'll be amazed at the progress you'll make toward your goal!

Here's my challenge to you: Wherever you have your affirmation written down, add the four words from today's success lesson to that piece of paper. Let them serve as inspiration to keep going when you face challenges along the way.

Dream, Believe, Dare, Do!

And, as we continue along on our journey together, always re-member: *I believe in you!*

LESSON 10:

One Healthy Choice After Another

Have you ever noticed how one good decision seems to lead to another?

The same can be said of bad decisions as well.

That's really what led us to being overweight, isn't it? It didn't happen overnight. Instead, it was a series of poor nutritional choices that led us to where we are today.

Now, I don't know *your* particular story, but I know that most of our stories go something like this:

At some point, we started eating and drinking more calories than we were burning off each day.

- This may have been during an extremely stressful time in our lives.
- It could have been during our carefree college days.
- Or it might have happened when we finally got out on our own and started deciding for ourselves what we would eat.

However we got there, this gradual accumulation of empty calories added up over time and turned into extra pounds that we started carrying around.

Just a few at first, a slight shift on the scale. No big deal. But a failure to adjust after this initial increase allowed the trend to continue.

Fast forward a few years and our small bad dietary decisions have resulted in weight gain and an unhealthy lifestyle. Our clothes are snug, we don't like the way we look, and we don't even bother stepping on the scale anymore.

*It's like the opposite of compound interest. Instead of small investments paying off and resulting in a nest egg, we end up with a body we don't like and an emotional bank account that's way overdrawn.

So, what do we do?

It starts with one good choice. That's all it takes. One positive decision in terms of your diet and your health can turn everything around.

It could be a subtle decision to eat less at each meal or to drink more water. Or it could be a major decision to lose 20 plus pounds or get back in shape.

If you'll make the decision to start on these paths and then make one healthy choice after another, you'll start to see how the same compounding effect that left you overweight and unhealthy can start to work *for you* instead.

Fewer calories plus more water and exercise quickly adds up in your favor and you'll start to see those excess pounds drop off as you discover a happier healthier lifestyle.

The choice is yours.

SUCCESS LESSON 10:

Your Secret Life

Have you seen the movie "The Secret Life of Walter Mitty?" (The one that stars Ben Stiller, not the weird 1947 version).

It's one of my favorite movies for many reasons, but one of the biggest reasons I love it is because it's the perfect story of how one choice can change everything in our lives for the better.

In the movie, Ben Stiller plays Walter, a man who gave up his dreams of travel and adventure to lead a responsible life after his father's death.

When we meet Walter, he's introduced as an extremely organized man. He's tedious when it comes to details. Everything in his life is about avoiding risk and the unknown.

Then, when an important photo negative goes missing (and his job is on the line) Walter embarks on a mission to track down the photographer and retrieve the negative.

From there, we watch as Walter flies to Greenland, jumps from a helicopter, fights a shark, journeys to an erupting volcano, and beyond...

After going on this journey, he emerges as a changed man. He's more confident, he's happier, his physical appearance even changes, and he gets the girl of his dreams/daydreams…

All because of his choice to take action and embark on an adventure.

You may not have realized it when you purchased this book, but you're on an adventure too!

- It's a journey to find the life of your dreams.
- A mission to find the future you long for.
- A quest to find a happier, healthier tomorrow.

It all started when you took a chance and bought this book. Now you just have to *stick with it* one day at a time, and who knows where you might end up!

*You see, far too many of us spend the better part of our lives daydreaming about a future that seems too good to be true, so we never set out on the adventure that would bring those dreams to life.

Instead, we live quiet, normal lives without real meaning or purpose.

All the while, our secret lives are there within us, longing to break free!

Does this sound too "pie in the sky?" It's not.

For proof, just think about the number of times you've felt a brief sensation of inspiration rise up within you.

Usually these bursts of inspiration are accompanied by "I wish" thoughts:

- I wish I could go there!
- I wish I could do *that*!
- I wish I could be (fill in the blank)!

The truth is you can! In fact, you're already on your way!

You purchased this book! You stepped out of your comfort zone! You dared to bring your dreams to life!

So, as we continue, don't ever lose sight of your Why. Keep it in front of you all the time. And, before you know it, it'll go from being your *secret life* to being the life you wake up to every day!

LESSON 11:

Discipline Makes the Difference

What makes the biggest difference in a person's success when it comes to reaching their weight-loss goals?

There are, admittedly, an almost infinite number of factors at play here, but the one I believe makes the biggest difference is discipline.

*Discipline turns "I wish I could" into "Here's how I'm going to…" and there's a huge difference between these two mindsets.

People with the first mindset wait for the stars to align perfectly so they can get started.

People with the second mindset take full responsibility for where they're at and decide to reach their goals *no matter what.*

Which type of person are you?

Now, what do I mean by disciplines?

I mean aligning your attitude and actions so they propel you toward your goal of losing weight. The result: You can say No to distractions because you've said Yes to your destination.

Think about it this way: Will one chocolate chunk cookie derail your entire diet? Not likely. But if you can say no to that cookie or a donut or a piece of cake, you're not only consuming fewer empty calories, you're building discipline.

You're saying No, because you've said Yes to something bigger.

These small victories will go a long way in helping you reach your ideal weight. And, once you get there, you can decide if you want to make sweets a part of your routine again.

Is discipline easy? Heck no! Saying no to ice cream the first time is almost painful. When your friend has a Blizzard treat and you have some fruit juice mixture in front of you, temptation will be at an all-time high.

But don't worry, Blizzards will still be there after you've reached your goal. And I guarantee you they'll taste sweeter when you're eating them as a reward for reaching your ideal weight than they ever did when you felt guilty for eating too much ice cream before your diet.

These small sacrifices make reaching your goal that much better.

You won't even think about all the ice cream you skipped when you've reached your weight-loss goal and you're looking and feeling great!

You may even want to save your ice cream money so you can use it to buy some smaller clothes!

SUCCESS LESSON 11:

Love and Discipline

Many times when the subject of discipline comes up, people are immediately turned off. And I can definitely understand that.

We tend to associate discipline with punishment.

It's perfectly natural. As children, when we did something bad, we got disciplined.

However, I want to take a look at discipline from a different angle.

What if instead of associating discipline with punishment, we started associating it with love?

Because, when it comes down to it, that's where most of the boundaries we set for our children come from, isn't it?

In order to protect them from harm, we set restrictions on where they can go and what they can do. Then, if they go beyond those boundaries, we discipline them because we love them too much to let them risk hurting themselves.

What's my point here?

*In order to reach our weight-loss goals, we have to discipline ourselves. Not as a punishment, but because we love ourselves too much to allow ourselves to fall back into unhealthy eating habits.

What does this look like on a practical level?

I think it means setting clear boundaries for ourselves. However, it's also important to frame those boundaries with the right mindset.

Instead of making a list of things we can't eat while we're on our diet and dwelling on the negative side of things, why not say, "Because I love the life that I've dreamed of, I'm choosing not to eat _______ right now."

Do you see the difference?

This kind of thinking shifts our focus from feeling deprived in the moment to feeling excited about the future.

Instead of thinking, "I can't eat bacon," think "Because I love the life of my dreams, I'm *choosing* not to eat bacon right now."

This is also where it's important to focus on what you *can* eat.

There's a whole world of foods for you to enjoy on a plant-based diet!

And not just the fruits and veggies that come to mind, there are also more and more meat alternatives available every day.

Just take a walk through the frozen section of your supermarket, and you'll see plant-based alternatives to many of your favorite foods.

So, decide today to tear up your "I can't eat" list.

Instead, start making a list of all of the plant-based foods you love, and then rotate through the list to keep things fresh! (Sorry, bad pun).

But seriously, get out there and try out some new plant-based recipes. You'll be amazed at the possibilities!

And, for those of you who are still bitter about me mentioning bacon above, here's a fun fact: McCormick's Bac'n Pieces don't technically have any meat in them, so feel free to sprinkle them on any plant-based foods you like!

LESSON 12:

Grocery Shopping 101

Let me start by saying I can't promise that you'll hear anything new in this lesson.

Instead, I want to share some insights that have been extremely helpful for me on my diet journey. I believe they'll help guide you to diet success as well!

My first piece of advice is an oldie but a goodie, "Don't shop hungry."

While this is important for people who aren't on a plant-based diet, it's absolutely *essential* when you're trying to lose weight.

Shopping hungry can lead to all kinds of unhelpful foods ending up in your cart, and then in your pantry. So, be sure to grab a healthy snack before heading out to the store!

My next piece of advice is also a classic, "Make a list."

It's so much easier to avoid impulse-buying when you go in with a list.

- Start by making a list of the plant-based meals you're planning to eat for the coming week.
- Then, write out a detailed list of what you'll need for each meal before you head to the store.
- Once you get to the store, stick to your list.

Another thing that helps is moving quickly past the sections with products you're not eating.

That means driving your cart right past the deli and bypassing the ice cream aisle altogether. Then move right on past the milk and skip the sweets too.

If you want to wave to them and tell them you miss them on your way past, I understand.

Here are a couple other options:

- If your budget allows, you may want to look at having your groceries delivered. That way you can bypass the grocery store altogether.
- Or, since you're making a list anyway, you may want to order online and then just go pick up your groceries.

The key is to find a method that helps you protect the progress you've made.

If you're an impulsive person, take steps to make sure you don't load your cart with foods that could set you back.

If you're a fairly disciplined person, you can probably wander the whole store and be fine.

Just be sure to recognize how you're wired and plan accordingly.

Remember to let your Why be your guide, even while you're grocery shopping. This will help you say No to unhealthy food choices because you've said Yes to your vision of the future.

Is that vision worth trading for a carton of ice cream? I don't think so!

SUCCESS LESSON 12:

Making A Meal Plan

When it comes to making a meal plan, your best bet is to keep it as simple as possible.

- First, get a blank piece of paper.
- Then, divide the paper into seven columns.
- Next, write out the days of the week from Monday through Sunday at the top of each of the seven columns.
- Now, divide each column into three sections and label them Breakfast, Lunch, and Dinner.

That's the framework for your weekly meal plan. From there, just fill in each of the meals with your favorite plant-based foods.

While there are a few different models available for plant-based eating, they tend to be fairly similar.

The two that make the most sense to me are the Food Triangle and the Plant-Based/Vegan Food Pyramid.

In the Food Triangle, you have three main categories:

- In the top circle, you have leafy greens, cruciferous vegetables, stems, bulbs, and mushrooms.
- The bottom left circle contains all of the animal foods: meat, eggs, dairy, poultry, fish, and shellfish.

- The bottom right circle contains plant foods: fruits, cereals, legumes, and starchy vegetables.
- Beside the plant foods circle is a smaller circle with nuts and seeds.

The emphasis in this model is to *eat on the right side of the triangle.*

Plant-Based/Vegan Food Pyramids can differ slightly, but generally have a similar emphasis to the Triangle.

- The bottom tier is made up of fruits (apples, oranges, bananas, grapes) on one side and vegetables (sweet potatoes, carrots, cucumbers) on the other.
- The next level contains leafy greens (spinach, broccoli, and kale) on one side and legumes (beans, peas, and lentils) on the other.
- Then it moves up to whole grains (oats, brown rice, whole grain pasta/tortillas, quinoa).
- At the top, you have whole foods that are high in fat (avocados, nuts, seeds, and soy-based substitutes for meat and dairy products).

The point of the Pyramid is to show that you want to eat more of the foods on the lower levels and be careful not to overdo the high fat foods on the top level.

In the end, these are just models. You can follow them, or simply use them as a rough idea of where to start.

The point in sharing these models is simply to give you some options to look at when you're considering how to fill in your meal plan. Ultimately, you'll want to tailor your plan to your own tastes.

My own meal plan featured a lot of bean and rice burritos on whole wheat tortillas, salads, fruit, and a plant-based bachelor's best friend: frozen vegetables you can steam in the microwave!

Okay, so now it's your turn, go ahead and fill in your meal plan. Remember to have fun, and don't be afraid to fill in something new and exciting once in a while!

You might just end up liking soy milk, vegan sausage, bean burgers, or whole wheat pasta or tortillas.

LESSON 13:

How to Survive Eating Out

Eating out is an everyday choice/routine for many people. It's faster, it's simpler, and it's more convenient to let someone else do the cooking.

I get it, I really do.

*Here's a hard truth: The people working at the restaurants you go to don't care about your health.

Do they want to hurt you? No.

If you and other people stopped coming in, they wouldn't have a job.

But this doesn't mean they have your best interests in mind when they're serving you.

You can walk into your local super buffet 365 days a year, and they'll keep taking your money and handing you a tray. It keeps them in business.

In fact, in a strange way, their customers' obesity is their job security.

Kind of sad, isn't it?

Anyway, now that you know the servers, fry cooks, and other workers aren't your friends, what's my point?

My point is that *you* have to have your best interests at heart when it comes to eating out.

Your friends and family may or may not have your diet in mind when they pick out a restaurant. So, you have to be prepared to respond in one of these ways:

1. Research that restaurant's menu to see what healthy meal options they have there. Then make the best choice you possibly can. It may be a salad or just a fruit cup.

   That's okay, just go and enjoy the time with the people you care about.

   It's amazing how much more enjoyable a meal can be when you're focused on fellowship instead of food.

   This leads us to response number two.

2. Don't eat.

   Sounds strange, right? It's really not.

   Just go along and hang out. Have fun spending time with your peeps. Use it as an opportunity to have some really good discussions about how everyone's doing and what's really going on in their lives.

3. Say No to going out.

   If you're not sure you can resist the temptation to go out and overeat, then staying home and eating well may be your best option.

   It's better to pass on an unhealthy choice than to fill up on food you'll regret eating.

My personal recommendation: Keep some granola bars or healthy snacks in your car or purse or briefcase or backpack.

If you get invited somewhere you know you'll be tempted to eat an unhealthy meal, eat your snack beforehand, then enjoy the time with your friends and eat a healthy meal after.

SUCCESS LESSON 13:

Turning Mealtime into Quality Time

I'm going to go into this idea a little further for a few minutes because this subject is one that's close to my heart, and because it's an area I often fall short in.

For so many of us, when we get together with friends or family for a meal, the focus is on the food.
Or, worse yet, our focus may be somewhere else entirely.

In this digital age, it's not uncommon to see a group of friends eating out "together." Only they're not really together, are they?

Sure, they're sitting at the same table. They're eating nearby each other. But they're not *connecting*. They're not really experiencing *togetherness* as it's meant to be.

That's where *you* come in.

The next time you go out to eat with friends or family members, *decide that you're going to pass on eating for that meal.*

(I know it sounds odd, but stick with me here).

Before you meet up for the meal, figure out who's going to be there, and write out some meaningful questions to ask each of them.

Then spend the entire meal, from the time you sit down to the time you head out, asking those questions and *really listening* to their responses.

- Ask about their day.
- Ask about their dreams.
- Ask about the dilemmas they're facing in life.
- Ask and then listen *intently*.

Somewhere along the way, we began to shift our focus from enjoying each other's company to entertaining our taste buds while people we care about sit nearby.

Let's change it up.

Be the first person to silence your cell phone at the table, look into the eyes of the person across from you, and ask them, "How are you *really* doing?"

And then see how the people you love come to life when they know that someone's *truly* listening to them.

LESSON 14:

To Cheat or Not to Cheat?

That is the question.

Many diets allow you a "cheat day" once a week when you can eat whatever you want. That way, you can splurge on carbs or calories or cupcakes and get it all out of your system in a single day.

Then you just go back to your regularly scheduled meal plan the next day.

*I'm *not* a fan.

Here are my reasons why:

1. On a plant-based diet, your goal is to limit the number of empty calories you take in. If you've done well all the way through the week and then you take in four times as many calories in one day, you're basically undoing all your hard work.

2. Your stomach is stretchy. That's probably not the technical term, but you know what I mean.

   Our goal is to get you eating today the way you want to be eating when you're at your ideal weight. That means your portion sizes should be decreasing as you go along.

Your stomach will adjust over time, and it'll take less food for you to feel full.

Eating a ton in one day sabotages your efforts in this area.

3. Yuck! What goes in must come out. 'Nough said.

Does that mean you should never reward yourself in *any way*?

Not at all.

But do it in a way that won't set you back or open the door for you to go back to bad habits.

What could this look like?

Let's say a family member doesn't know (or forgets) about your diet and sends you a box full of truffles... *burn them*!

No, not really.

Here's what I did when this happened to me: I ate a couple over a one-week period. Then, the first Christmas party I attended, I took the rest and gave them away.

Problem solved.

We need rewards for our good habits. The problem is that many of us have been raised to equate rewards for our accomplishments with food.

Like ice cream after a baseball game.

But what if you do something different?

What if the next time you have a great week on your diet, you take yourself shopping instead?

You can pick up a nice shirt you hope to shrink into, buy a book on motivation or success, or take yourself out to a movie.

The key is to keep moving forward, and *cheat days cost too much*.

SUCCESS LESSON 14:

Your New Mantra

"**I** can eat whatever I want, but I'm choosing to follow a plant-based diet."

Here's the deal, your inner child is a little rascal. He or she is like a little spoiled three-year-old who hates being told No. So, you need to outsmart him or her.

What do I mean by that?

I mean that if you tell yourself, "I can't eat anything sugary or any meat or have any dairy products," you'll immediately start *wanting* those things.

You'll notice them everywhere you go, and you'll feel guilty if you ever give in and eat them.

Instead, I recommend that you adopt this slogan and mindset: "I can eat whatever I want, but I'm *choosing* to follow a plant-based diet because (insert your Why here)."

How does this help?

- First, it gets rid of the "I can't" mindset that causes psychological tension inside of you.

- Second, you acknowledge that eating something off-diet isn't the end of the world.

> Does it help? No. But it won't make or break your diet either.

- Third, the last part keeps you focused on your goal.

  Think back to your Why…

  "Because I really want to be able to play with my kids/grandkids" or "Because I want to prove to myself that I can lose the weight and keep it off."

*Remember, keeping your motivation for losing the weight at the front of your mind will help you say No to temptations because you've said Yes to your goal.

Your diet is your own.

I can't come and check your fridge to see if you're eating meat or dairy products.

I can make recommendations, but I can't enforce them.

How you proceed is up to you.

I can tell you that the mindset/mantra above served me well on my own journey—especially when well-meaning friends would ask questions like, "Can you have *this*? What about *that?*"

Rather than try to explain what was or wasn't "allowed" on my diet, I would just remind them, "I can eat whatever I want…"

Just make sure you don't use this as an excuse to stray back into unhealthy habits. A piece of garlic toast won't ruin your diet, but a bowl of spaghetti with meat sauce is pushing it.

Think about our road trip analogy again: You can stop to see a tourist attraction here and there, but don't take up residence!

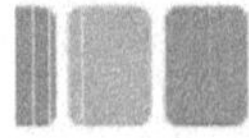

Plant-Based Diet Success

Week 3: Staying Focused

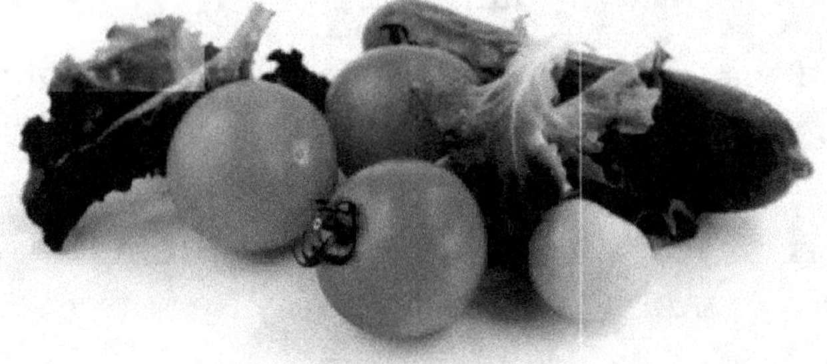

LESSON 15:

Halfway There!

You're now halfway into this book!

My hope is that you're applying the principles I've been sharing with you, and that they're starting to pay off as you find yourself weighing less and feeling better.

What kind of results should you be seeing?

This will vary from person to person. Some people might lose 14 pounds in 14 days. Others may only lose a pound a week. The important thing is that you get the scale moving in the right direction.

Remember, this isn't an overnight miracle diet. It's a lifestyle change based on making one good choice after another until you reach your ideal weight and take hold of the reason you started losing weight to begin with. Your Why!

The principles work if you work the principles. It's as true in dieting as it is in any other area of your life. If you learn to discipline yourself and pursue healthy habits each and every day, you'll start to see results.

Is this always easy? Not at all!

Change is challenging.

Our minds like routine. In fact, we're wired to run on autopilot. One of the ways we see this is when we drive the same route over and over again day after day. We can get to the point where we can't even remember that morning's commute.

The great thing about this is that healthy dietary choices can become second nature as well! You may start out having to intentionally seek out healthy snacks and fight against the urge to grab something sweet and fattening instead.

But, eventually, you'll find that it really isn't all that hard to pass on dessert as your goal starts to come into view. And the closer it gets, the more your momentum builds until you end up sprinting to the finish line!

Does that sound impossible from where you're at? Trust me, it's not.

Remember, I've been there too.

I spent years overweight and unhealthy. And I rode the roller-coaster of trying to lose weight without a solid plan.

This diet helped me to break that cycle, and I hope it's helping you to do the same.

Wherever you're at today, keep going on this plan. I know first-hand that it can *literally* change your life. And that's why you're here, right? Because you want the life you've always dreamed of.

It's yours, if you just keep going!

SUCCESS LESSON 15:

Taking Action to Achieve Your Dreams

One of the most powerful books I've come across in my personal development journey is You²: A High Velocity Formula for Multiplying Your Personal Effectiveness in Quantum Leaps by Price Pritchett, PH.D.

In one of my favorite chapters of this short (but powerful) book, he shares this insight:

> "You've dreamed many dreams that were yours for the taking.
>
> In fact, almost all of them were well within your reach.
> Even now, most of what you dream can be yours.
> The simple secret is the seeking...
> Consider this—the dreams you have realized in life are those which you actively sought. That which you have achieved is what you decided to go for in one way or another. You can 'think positively' all day long, all year, but positive action is what counts."

Pretty incredible stuff, right? Every page of the book is packed with gems like that, so be sure to pick up a copy ASAP!

With all of that being said, how are you doing in terms of taking action?

- Are you reading over your weight loss affirmation

every day?
- Are you planning out your meals ahead of time?
- Are you staying disciplined and only eating plant-based foods?

Following these small steps consistently is the key to achieving your weight-loss goals.

You've already made the quantum leap out of the unhealthy lifestyle you were leading before. You've made the decision to leave behind the eating habits that were keeping you unhealthy and unhappy.

Now you just have to keep taking action to move toward your dream of a happier, healthier life!

Before we launch into the second half of this book, I just want you to know that I'm so happy you're here! I'm proud of the progress you've made so far! And I'm excited for the results you'll see as you keep moving forward on your journey to diet success!

LESSON 16:

Traps and Temptations

You'll be amazed what looks appetizing to you in the middle of a craving.

You've heard about the pregnant woman who craves pickles and ice cream, right?

On this diet, you may get some crazy cravings too.

- Desserts you never liked before will start calling out to you.
- Candy you would've passed up is now begging for you to eat it.
- And don't be surprised if coworkers who've never offered to share anything with you the entire time you've worked together start offering you sweets out of nowhere.

It happens. And, while you can't always *control* your cravings, you can *combat* them.

Here are a few things you can do:

1. <u>Say "No, thank you."</u> - Does this seem rude? It isn't.

   You can thank them for offering it to you. You can let them know you appreciate them thinking of you. But you're not obligated to guzzle every sweet drink or devour every Christmas cookie people shove at you.

Think of it this way: if you offered them something and they said they were on a diet, would you be offended? Of course not! You'd keep your sweets to yourself, commend them on their self-control, and wish them well.

So, with that in mind, why would you be obligated to indulge in whatever *they're offering you*? That's right, you're not.

Just say No, or "No, thank you."

2. <u>Eat some fruit or another healthy sweet snack</u>- When your brain's telling you, "Hey, we need something sweet *now!*" First, realize that's not true. You'll never *need* sweets to survive. Second, as a way of appeasing your brain, eat something sweet...

   Just make sure it's healthy. It's better to eat a small healthy snack than starve yourself or eat something that's going to set you back.

Don't even open that door.

Instead, know ahead of time that these cravings will come and keep snacks on-hand for just such a situation. Then you can feel good about turning down the candy, donuts, or piece of cake, all while continuing on toward your goal.

Again, please believe me when I say these moments *will* come.

Be ready to make good choices when they do. And remember, these temptations may very well come from people who love you the most.

SUCCESS LESSON 16:

The Power of F.O.C.U.S.

I can't remember exactly where I ran across this acronym, but the lesson itself has stuck with me ever since I read it.

You see, for many of us, our problem is not a lack of desire.

- We *want* to lose weight.
- We *want* to get into shape.
- We *want* to live happier, healthier lives.
- And we *want* to achieve our dreams.

So, if the problem isn't with our desires, what is it?

*For many of us, the issue is a lack of focus.

Our lives get so hectic that we simply lose sight of our goals and dreams.

You've probably used all of the same excuses I have:

- "I'm so busy…"
- "I'm so tired…"
- "It's just easier to…"

In the end, those excuses are just an easy way to justify the behaviors that are holding us back from reaching our goals.

However, it's amazing what can happen when we master the power of F.O.C.U.S. That stands for: Follow One Course Until

Successful.

This applies to any goals that we set for our lives, but it's especially important when it comes to dieting.

How many people do you know who start one project after another (or one *diet* after another), but never really seem to get any of them *done*?

I know I've been one of those people in the past.

The point here *isn't* to make you feel guilty, it's to encourage you to stay the course.

Keep going on your plant-based diet. Stick with it even through the challenges, mishaps, or temptations that are sure to come up along the way.

It's entirely possible that your emotions may start to get the best of you, and you'll begin to doubt that your diet's working. This is where *a lot* of people simply give up.

Don't let that be *your* story!

Instead, remember that success often only comes on the other side of incredible obstacles. And success on your diet journey is no different.

So, on those tough days, hold onto these three things:

1. The Why you chose when you started your diet.
2. The fact that if you're eating less and exercising more, the weight *will* come off.
3. And this question: What it will make of you to see this journey through to the end?

For me, reaching my weight-loss goal was a much-needed success. Being human, and having more than my fair share of ups and downs along the way, I *really* needed a win.

The plant-based diet gave me that win, and the lessons I learned along the way have given me the courage to pursue some of the biggest goals I've ever had in my life- like writing this book!

My hope is that seeing this diet through to the end, reaching your ideal weight, and bringing *your Why* to life will do the same thing for you.

And remember, I'll be here with you every step of the way!

LESSON 17:

Why Motivation Matters

Let's talk a little more about why motivation is so important.

We already discussed why finding and naming your Why is an essential part of reaching your weight-loss goals, but I think this subject is worth revisiting.

You see, we ended up overweight and unhappy with our bodies for a reason.

Sometimes that reason is biological.

For most of us, our reason was much more *psychological.*

*Somewhere along the way, we lost sight of our reason to stay fit and healthy.

After reaching this point, we started making one bad diet choice after another, until we got where we are today.

What did these choices look like?

- Burger after burger
- Soda after soda
- Beer after beer
- Donut after donut
- Candy bar after candy bar

If you turned to one (or more) of these things when you were having a bad day, you're not alone. Many of us fall into the trap of turning to food for comfort when we lose sight of our motivation for reaching our goals in life.

Don't you *dare* beat yourself up over this!

For many of us, the habit of numbing ourselves with food was triggered by a traumatic event that left us devastated. And over-eating seemed like the least harmful vice we could turn to in order to cope with that situation.

Please hear me when I say that ending up in this situation doesn't make you weak or bad or shameful or any of the other negative things you might have called yourself along the way.

It just makes you *human*.

And that's a *good thing*!

Why?

Because as humans, we can accomplish almost anything we set our minds to—*with the proper motivation.*

What does this process look like?

1. Take full responsibility for where you're at. One way or another, our choices led us to where we are today. The good news is: *better choices can lead us right back out of here.*

2. Change your identity. You have to kill off all of your "I *justs*."

   As in:
   "I *just* can't help it."
   "I *just* eat when I'm stressed."
   "I *just* need a few drinks to unwind."
   "I *just* (insert destructive or counterproductive habit) when I'm (insert excuse)."

Quit it!

When we use phrases like these, we're playing the victim and giving ourselves permission to stay the same because, "It's *just* who I am."

That's nonsense!

For the most part, *we are who we've decided to become.* In this way, our present health is the natural result of our dietary decisions.

Fortunately, if our decisions have led us to the point of being overweight, we can decide to become a physically fit and healthy person *instead.*

Making this decision is the Yes that will help you say No to future bad diet choices.

And it's also the decision that will lead you back to a life of self-confidence, joy, and achieving all your goals and dreams!

Feeling motivated yet?

Awesome! Let's keep going.

You've got this!

SUCCESS LESSON 17:

Your Bigger Picture

If you haven't noticed, Jack Canfield is one of my favorite success coaches and authors.

For those who are new to Jack's teaching, be sure to read his book <u>The Success Principles: How to Get from Where You Are to Where You Want to Be</u> (which he co-authored with Janet Switzer).

Honestly, it'll change your life, so go add it to your Wish List on Amazon or Audible! (I highly recommend the 10th Anniversary Edition).

One of the practices Jack recommends is writing out your goals for each of these seven major areas of your life:

Financial Goals| Career/Business Goals
Free Time/Family Time Goals
Health/Appearance Goals| Relationship Goals
Personal Growth Goals
Making A Difference/Legacy Goals

So, as long as we're on the subject of motivation, why not go ahead and write out your own goals for these seven areas?

Jack sets three goals in each area per year, for a total of 21 goals.

You may just want to start with one for each category, or you may be able to come up with all 21 right now.

Again, think back to your Why, and be sure to work that into your Health/Appearance Goals.

Remember, they're *your* goals, so dream big!

Think about this question for a moment: If you could have your life *exactly* the way you want it one year from now, what would it look like?

Go ahead and close your eyes and picture your ideal life for a few moments.

*Seriously, go ahead.

Okay, now that you have a clearer picture of your dream life, start filling in your Goals List.

(Insert semi-awkward silence here while you write out your goals).

What should you do with your list once you complete it?

Many people will simply set their list aside or throw it away.

My advice: Keep it where you can see it. Then, when you go over your weight loss affirmation, read through your goals list as well.

To get the most out of this practice, write your goals out as though you've already accomplished them.

Remember the formula: "I'm so happy and grateful I'm enjoying <u>(insert your completed goal)</u>!"

Just like with your affirmation, be sure to trace your finger over your goals as you read them, to help get your subconscious brain working on them too.

Then take time to picture your goals as already accomplished and *feel the feelings* you'll feel when you really do bring all your dreams to life.

I understand that it feels a little silly at first (trust me).

But I also know that repeating this one practice a few times a day can lead to incredible results and a more inspired life!

So, try it out.

What've you got to lose?

*Want to take this exercise to the next level? Share your goals with a close friend or family member. Remember, writing out your goals *and* sharing them with someone else *dramatically increases your likelihood of achieving them!*

LESSON 18:

The Power of Persistence

You have to decide early on that you'll do whatever it takes to reach your weight-loss goal. Otherwise, something will come along and derail your diet.

Developing a strong sense of persistence (also known as grit or stick-to-itiveness) will greatly improve your chances of success.

Think about it this way: If you're a parent and one of your kids goes missing in a busy store, you do whatever it takes to find them. You don't stop looking because you're tired, or it's "just too hard," you keep searching until they're back in your arms again!

Is the future you've pictured any less important to you?

What would you sacrifice to have the life you've dreamed of?

It could cost you money, delayed gratification, time, energy, comfort, and many other things.

Are you ready to make those sacrifices?

Ask yourself: Is losing weight something you'd *like* to do, or is it something you believe you *must* do?

As John Assaraf would ask, "Are you interested or *committed*? If you're interested, you'll do what's convenient. If you're committed, you'll do whatever it takes!"

Some of you may have *literally* been told that your life depends on you losing weight. For the rest of us, the hope of a better future can be a major motivator.

Persistence means getting up when you fall. It means starting the next day with renewed vigor after a night of unhealthy eating. It means skipping seconds on your favorite foods and saying No to incredible desserts. And it means doing all of this without an immediate reward.

As I said before, it's not easy. That's why so many people give up and decide they're "never going to lose" all their extra weight.

Again, please don't let that be *your* story.

Yes, dieting can be difficult, but it's also worth it!

Will you hit walls or plateau along the way at different times? It's possible.

Persistence is most essential at times like these!

You may have to cut back even more on the number of calories you're eating.

You may have to spend more time walking or exercising.

At times like these, *keep your Why in the front of your mind.*

- If you're losing weight so you can be more active in your kids' or grandkids' lives, keep their picture where you can see it.
- If you're trying to slim down and fit into your old jeans, keep them out in the open.
- If you're seeking to regain self-confidence, hold onto a picture from the time in your life when you felt most vibrant and passionate!

These reminders of what you're working towards will help you stay strong in the hard times.

And remember to keep track of the progress you've made up to this point. Even if you're not losing weight as quickly as you'd like.

As long as you're making healthier choices each and every day, take time to celebrate every small victory!

SUCCESS LESSON 18:

The Positive Change Cycle

Any time we launch into a new endeavor (a new job, a new diet, a new habit, etc.), we're going to run into the tension that comes with changing our lives.

It's so common that psychologists have developed the Positive Change Cycle to illustrate the process all of us go through as we seek to improve our lives.

In fact, you've probably seen this cycle play out in your own life along the way.

Here are the five steps:

- Uninformed Optimism
- Informed Pessimism
- Crisis of Means
- Informed Optimism
- Completion

Here's how the Cycle plays out:

1. Uninformed Optimism- We tend to launch into new experiences with a lot of passion and enthusiasm. For example, if you've ever gone skiing and watched a friend who's fairly experienced glide down the slope with ease, it

looks pretty simple, right?

Watching them gives us a sense of uninformed optimism. "I can do that!" we think…

2. Informed Pessimism- This is the part where we fall on our butt (or worse). We strap on our skis, grab our poles, and get ready to glide down the hill (just like our friend did). Then we fall on our face, spit out some snow, and wonder how in the world we ever let them talk us into strapping these devices of death onto our ski boots!

This leads us to the most important part of the process.

3. The Crisis of Means- This is the middle of the process. The point of decision. Do we keep going and try again, or do we drag our skis back up the slope and turn them in?

If you're like me, you've had moments in your life where you've pushed through, and you've had moments where you gave up. This is usually when that happens.

You've realized that it's not going to be as easy as it looked. You're going to have to gain new skills and be willing to fail before you get better. And you have to decide if the end result is worth the persistence required to get there.

4. Informed Optimism- Luckily, for many of us, our desire to succeed overrides our pessimism, and we get back up. We go back to the top of the hill, ask our friend to show us how it's done, and then give the bunny slope another go.

Now we know what we're up against, and we're ready to face the challenge. We may not make it the second time, the third time, or even the fifteenth time, but we're determined to learn how to ski, and nothing's going to stop us!

5. Completion- This is where things get really good! We've stuck it out and honed our skills. We've weathered the ups and downs (literally), and now it's smooth sailing.

It's around this time that we have our first perfect (or near-perfect) run, and it's all worth it!

Not only that, but we're also in a position to share what we've learned with others and help them find success!

Regardless of where you're at in the Positive Change Cycle with your diet, the key thing I want you to take away from this lesson is that just by continuing to work through this course you're on your way to success!

You may be experiencing fantastic results, or they may be a little slower in coming than you would've hoped, but you're still here! You're sticking with it, and that's fantastic!

Keep coming back and learning more.

Keep on following along and putting what you're learning into action- even on the days when it's hard!

And, one of these days, I look forward to hearing your Success Story!

LESSON 19:

Don't Let Guilt Get You Down

On the off chance that your diet journey's not going precisely like you thought it would, I wanted to share a lesson to help you get back on track.

Let's face it: *No weight-loss plan goes exactly the way we hope it will.* There are twists and turns and detours we have to face all along the way. Some of these we navigate successfully, others we don't.

*The key to success is not letting these things deter you from moving forward—especially when it comes to guilt.

Guilt can show up in any number of ways on your weight-loss journey. It can come in the form of feeling guilty for letting yourself get as heavy as you have. It can come if you make a bad meal choice or binge on snack cakes or indulge in a dessert that's not in your best interest.

Whatever scenario prompts you to feel guilty, the key is not to let it overwhelm you. This is one reason I encourage the mantra I mentioned before, because it cuts you some slack and keeps guilt from coming in.

But let's say that you *really* screw up.

I mean you just completely let yourself go and you go back to the way you were eating before starting your diet. You binge on all your favorite fatty foods for a week and you're disgusted with yourself.

Shouldn't you feel guilty?

Shouldn't you wallow in your bad choices?

You certainly have that option, but let me ask you this question: If your best friend were on a diet and *they* had a really bad week, what would you say to them?

- Would you tell them to just give up?
- Would you rub their nose in their bad choices and call them a failure?
- Would you make them feel guilty and encourage them to dwell on that guilt the rest of their lives?

No way!

- You would pick them back up, dust them off, and encourage them to keep going.
- You would tell them you believe in them and you know they can do this!
- You would tell them one bad week doesn't mean they should just give up.
- And you would tell them *you're not giving up on them that easily!*

*Give yourself the same grace you'd give to your best friend!

If you're coming to this lesson after getting sidetracked on your diet for a while, pick yourself up, dust yourself off, and get back on track.

Refocus on your Why and start moving forward again.

You can still do this!

I *still* believe in you. And no snags you hit along the way could change that!

SUCCESS LESSON 19:

Facing the Brick Walls

Another one of my favorite books is The Last Lecture by Randy Pausch. Randy was a computer science professor at Carnegie Mellon University whose struggle with terminal cancer led him to think about the lessons and stories he wanted to leave behind for his children.

He initially shared these lessons in a lecture at the university called "Really Achieving Your Childhood Dreams," and then he also put them into a book with the help of Jeffrey Zaslow.

If you haven't watched the lecture or read the book, you should check them out.

One of the lessons Randy shared which stood out to me the most was a lesson about brick walls. Thinking back to a time when he applied for an internship with Walt Disney Imagineering (and was initially rejected), he said, "...that was a bit of a setback. But remember, the brick walls are there for a reason. *The brick walls are not there to keep us out. The brick walls are there to give us a chance to show how badly we want something.* Because the brick walls are there to stop the people who don't want it badly enough. They're there to stop the *other* people."

Sometimes dieting can feel like a series of brick walls.

Maybe you've had one of these experiences with a diet in the past:

- You change your eating habits, but don't see any results.
- You add exercise to your routine, and you *gain* a couple pounds.
- You lose several pounds, but then you plateau, and it seems impossible to make any more progress.
- Or maybe you reached your goal, but then gained all the weight back.

On an emotional level, these scenarios can all feel like running full force into a brick wall.

The fact is: brick walls happen in life.

- In diets.
- In careers.
- In relationships.

The question isn't "Will I hit a brick wall?" It's "What do I do *when* I hit a brick wall?"

Think about it: How many people hit a snag in their diet and just give up?

The honest answer is probably *most*.

Consider the number of people who make a new year's resolution to lose weight and then give up by Valentine's Day.

It's simply easier *not to try*.

Change is difficult, especially when it involves major shifts in your routine or your way of thinking.

It's easier to just settle for the way things are, even if you're miserable.

Randy's quote is a great way to keep these brick walls in perspective.

When it comes down to it, how badly do you want the life of your dreams?

Are you willing to find a way over, around, or through the brick wall? Or will you give up and turn around like so many people?

I chose the tagline "A fun and simple way to lose weight and feel great- for life" because I honestly believe that a plant-based diet is just that. However, that doesn't mean you might not hit a brick wall (or three) along the way.

My hope is that, if you *do* hit a brick wall, you'll look for a way past it.

Don't run away from it. Instead, think of a way to overcome it.

You see, a lot of people stop themselves *before they even get started*. They think, "What if I try a new diet and it doesn't work?"

That's the negative side of "what if."

*I want you to look on the positive side:

- "What if this is the perfect diet for me?"
- "What if I can *finally* get rid of my baby weight?"
- "What if I lose the weight, and then help my (friend, husband, child) lose weight too?"

So, what do you say?

Wanna climb over some walls together?

Awesome! Let's keep going!

LESSON 20:

Swearing Off Sweets

"**A**re you serious?" You might be asking right now. Yes, and No.

Yes, I think you'll benefit greatly from stepping away from sweets for a while. No, I don't expect you to give them up forever.

Ultimately, if you can set sweets aside and get some perspective, you'll see they're just not worth the admiration you've been giving them.

Cookies, cakes, pies, candy, and ice cream are all loaded with sugar and empty calories, and they're at the heart of how most of us gained our unwanted weight. The same could be said of sugary sodas or drinks that are really desserts with a splash of coffee.

Is this an easy process? Nope.

I won't even pretend like it is.

There's a reason we turn to these foods when we're trying to feel better. Maybe it's the sugar rush we get or the sense of nostalgia some of these treats give us. Or maybe our taste buds are just crying out for entertainment.

Whatever the reason, the sweets must go. At least for a while.

Why? Because they're the nutritional opposite of everything this diet is trying to help you achieve. By eating lots of sweets, you're (at best) holding yourself back from reaching your ideal weight as quickly as possible. And (at worst) you're shooting yourself in the foot and destroying the possibility of ever reaching your goal.

Like we talked about before, sweets will still be there after you've reached your ideal weight. Ice cream isn't going away anytime soon. But for now, let it go.

Do a sugar detox and get it out of your system so you can move forward.

How do I recommend you do this? Start by clearing out all the sweets from your house.

Again, I realize you probably live with other people who won't appreciate this kind of purge, so you'll have to do one of two things:

1. Get them on board too.
2. Set aside a space in your pantry that's just for your snacks.

Once you've done that, stock your space with fruit and nuts or even organic fruit snacks—whatever healthy snacks you think might satisfy your sweet tooth and keep you on track.

Be sure to discipline yourself when you're eating out as well. Always pass on soda at the restaurant. If you need caffeine, get your fix with a caffeinated drink mix on the way there.

To use an illustration from Jack Canfield, trying to lose weight while continuing to eat sweets is like driving with your emergency brake on. It creates unnecessary tension and hinders your progress.

So, why not give up the sweets, release the brake, and increase your progress?

SUCCESS LESSON 20:

The Not-So-Sweet Life

If someone drinks alcohol to the point that it destroys their liver, we call them an alcoholic.

If someone uses drugs until they lose their job, their health, and their family we call them a drug addict.

But whereas saying "I'm an alcoholic" or "I'm a drug addict" are words that can silence a room. The phrase "I'm a sugar addict" often elicits little more than a chuckle.

Here's the deal: According to Addiction Center, "Some studies have suggested sugar is as addictive as *cocaine*."

According to their website on the subject (https://www.addictioncenter.com/drugs/sugar-addiction/), "...approximately 75% of Americans eat excess amounts of sugar, many of whom could be classified as having a sugar addiction."

When you take a second to really think about that, it kind of takes the fun out of being a sugar addict, doesn't it?

As long as we're getting real on the subject, isn't an addiction to sugar (or using food as a coping mechanism) really the one "socially acceptable" addiction out there?

And yet, the consequences can be just as severe as those of abusing drugs or alcohol.

It's possible to eat enough sugar to cause our weight to sky-rocket and even put our body in a pre-diabetic state.

Not only that, but *our children often follow in our footsteps when it comes to sugar addiction.* I mean, we would never hand them a crack pipe or a bottle of beer, we just let them binge on candy or keep the fridge stocked with soda for them.

Too harsh?

According to the CDC (https://www.cdc.gov/healthyschools/obesity/index.htm), "Data from 2015–2016 show that nearly 1 in 5 school-age children and young people aged 6 to 19 years in the United States has obesity."

One. In. Five.

Let's do something about all of this!

We have to be more careful about how we treat our bodies and the behaviors we model for our children. We have to show them there's a better, healthier way to live.

If you're like me, depression may be one of the reasons you've turned to food as a coping mechanism in the past. In some strange way, entertaining our taste buds or chasing a sugar rush can help to numb the pain of depression for a while (though it never does anything about our *actual* life issues).

Ironically, according to the Addiction Center site referenced above, using sugar as a coping mechanism, "…can damage self-esteem, cause feelings of helplessness, and lower self-worth, which in turn leads to more sugar consumption and a more severe addiction."

So, the very thing we turn to for comfort becomes its own kind of prison.

If sugar is still a major factor in your diet, it's time to cut it out.

To reuse an illustration from earlier in the book, trying to lose weight while consuming large amounts of sugar is like trying to run a race with a backpack full of bricks.

Instead, start looking for healthy foods to eat when your sweet tooth kicks in. Keep fruit on-hand for you and your kids to snack on.

Don't ever buy soda to put in your fridge. Make it off-limits in your house. If you get a craving for caffeine, get it from a zero-calorie drink mix you can put in your water.

When you think about your Why, does it only involve *you* being happier and healthier, or *do you picture the people around you being happier and healthier too?*

If so, kick sugar to the curb. You'll be amazed at how it'll springboard your weight-loss to new levels, and you'll be saving your family from the trap of sugar addiction at the same time!

On a related note, trying to launch into the future of your dreams while dwelling on your past can be just as self-defeating as harboring a sugar addiction.

Again, if depression has been a trap for you, I hope that you'll seek help in letting go of your past hurts and struggles. I know it can be extremely difficult.

Trust me, I'm as guilty as the next person when it comes to looking into the mirror and seeing only my scars, but *there's a better way for us to live.* A big part of that "better way" involves deciding that you want a happier, healthier life for yourself and believing that you deserve it.

If that's still a struggle for you; then, for now, just know that *I* believe it. And, rest assured that by working your way through this book, you're making the kinds of healthy choices that can turn your whole life around.

LESSON 21:

Drink More to Lose More

Would you believe that water can be one of your best resources when it comes to losing weight?

According to Doctor Michael Smith (Chief Medical Editor at WebMD), drinking more water "…means you'll eat fewer calories. You'll also benefit from a drop in saturated fat, sugar, sodium, and cholesterol."

Dr. Smith also points out that by drinking three extra cups of water a day, you can reduce your calorie intake by 205 calories. *You'd have to walk two and a half miles to burn that many calories!*

I don't know about you, but that's enough to keep me chugging water every day.

Think of it as your diet booster. Sure, you'll probably lose weight even if you just change up your eating habits, but why not use water to springboard you to success?

Take a minute to picture how the food you eat moves through your body. Would you rather have it flow through easily (like water), or move in a slow and sticky stream (like soda syrup)?

We've all heard the phrase, "You are what you eat." However, we don't always give as much thought to what we drink.

Now, some of you have been faithful in drinking water for years, and that's awesome!

I got into the habit of drinking Kool-Aid, soda, or juice with every meal from an early age, so this was a particularly hard habit for me to break.

Drinking more water has been one of the biggest pieces in my dieting success. By drinking water, I've been able to avoid at least 300 calories a day that I would have taken in otherwise. That's 9000 calories I'm avoiding over the course of a month. That's huge!

What has your calorie intake looked like?

- Maybe it was a glass of milk or a designer coffee in the morning.
- Then a soda and a free refill at lunch (that "free" refill added another 140+ calories).
- And maybe you had another soda or an alcoholic beverage at dinner.

These dietary choices could add over 500 calories to your day! And none of them are helping you reach your weight-loss goals.

If this has been your story, it's time to change it. Drastically.

I'm all for a serving of fruit juice in the morning. These calories are your friend.

Otherwise, cut out as many calories as you can.

Drink water everywhere you go, and try out those zero-calorie drink mixes you can put in your water to add flavor (and get your caffeine fix too).

*When the water starts dripping out of your ears, you've had enough. Otherwise, drink as much as you can. You'll be amazed at the difference drinking plenty of water will make in how you feel.

Drinking water can also be extremely helpful when it comes to dealing with hunger. If you're feeling hungry and you drink a bottle of water and the hunger goes away, it may be that you were really just misinterpreting a signal from your body that it was thirsty.

If you still feel hungry, you can always eat a healthy snack.

Don't let drinking calories derail you on your way to diet success. Cut out as many empty calories from drinks as you can, and be careful when you start to reintroduce them. This trap can hurt you just as much in the future as it has in the past.

Remember, when it comes to losing weight, every little bit helps. That includes cutting calories by drinking more water. And, as you can tell from Dr. Smith's comment above, a little bit goes a long way!

SUCCESS LESSON 21:

Compounding Your Results

When you start to think about making healthy choices (like drinking more water) as ways of investing in yourself, it puts these healthy habits in a new perspective.

Think about it, when you're first trying to lose weight and you have a goal of shedding (let's say) 50 pounds, losing a single pound doesn't feel like a huge victory.

Now, fast forward a few months and let's say you're within five pounds of your ideal weight. At this point, each pound is a tremendous accomplishment!

Does that make sense?

If not, consider those fractions in a food analogy:

1/50th of a pizza isn't much.

1/5th of a pizza is huge!

*My point is, when you dedicate yourself to making one healthy choice after another, the results aren't just cumulative, they're exponential!

Let's look at it a different way.

If you take $100 out of every paycheck and stuff it in your mattress, it'll definitely add up over time.

However, if you invest that same $100 a paycheck in a mutual fund and let compound interest go to work for you, the results are exponentially greater!

The truth is, making healthy choices can be a challenge—especially after years of living with unhealthy habits. But when you begin to practice one healthy choice after another, you start to build positive momentum, and you make your journey to diet success that much easier.

What do these choices look like?

You're probably making a lot of them already:

- Eating/drinking healthier
- Exercising more
- Setting goals
- Measuring results
- Practicing persistence
- Strengthening relationships
- Planning for success
- Building better habits

Each of the steps you've been taking since you started reading this book is like putting a dollar in your investment account. And, I can promise you this, if you keep investing in yourself each day (just like you have been) you're going to see a windfall of results in the days to come!

The most exciting part? Unlike investing in the stock market with all of its ups and downs, *the investments you make in yourself are guaranteed to pay off in the long run.*

What are these pay-offs?

- Increased energy
- Boosted self-confidence
- Better health
- A longer life
- More brainpower

- And any of the other results you're after!

So, keep making healthy choices.

And remember, you're not just saving for a rainy day, you're investing in the life of your dreams!

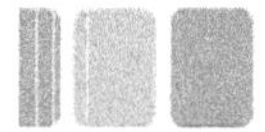

Plant-Based Diet Success
Week 4: Achieving Results

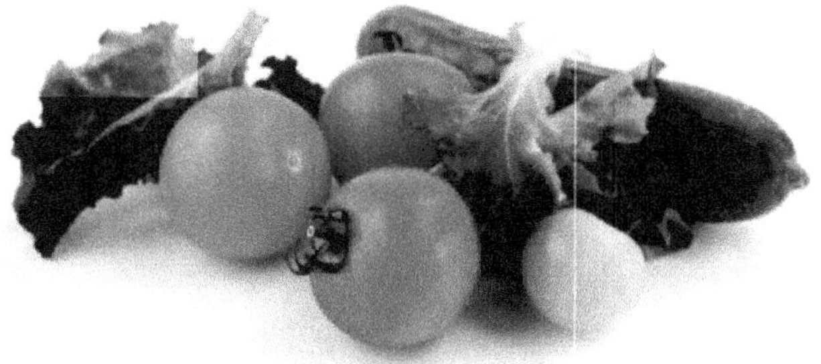

LESSON 22:

How to Avoid Snacking Screw-Ups

Have you ever had a "quick bite" turn into an awful binge?

I know I have. I've bet that I *could have just one chip* (like the commercial says), and lost that bet many times.

That's why I recommend snacking with a plan in mind.

- <u>First, make sure you only have access to healthy snacks</u>- this is the biggest part of the snacking battle. If you overeat on fruit, you'll probably be okay. At least it's better than eating a ton of snack cakes...

- <u>Second, have your snacking portions measured out ahead of time</u>. It's better if you can put them in Tupperware or a zip-lock bag (if they don't already come in small pouches).

This way, when you go looking for a snack, you know you're only going to eat your pre-measured portion.

This is extremely helpful when it comes to avoiding binge eating.

- <u>Third, give yourself *permission* to snack</u>.

In the past, you may have equated snacking with excess.

"I already had a meal, and now I'm eating a snack too!" you might have thought.

On a plant-based diet, snacks can be your best friend. This is because our goal is to drastically reduce your portion sizes and your calorie intake. That doesn't happen overnight.

We're basically reprogramming your body and your brain. And, as we mentioned before, if your inner child feels like they're being punished (or starved) he or she tends to act out.

So, don't be afraid to snack. I recommend eating a good breakfast and then having a mid-morning snack of nuts or fruit.

Eat your healthy lunch and then have a mid-afternoon snack. And, if you feel like you really need a snack after dinner, it's not life or death either.

Try to hold out until bedtime if you can, but don't feel bad for a single second if you need to eat a little more to get by.

Ultimately, having a snack plan saves you from going overboard if/when you get hungry after a meal. And, early on in this diet, there's a good chance that will happen.

But good discipline here will go a long way toward keeping you on track to reach your goals and get down to your ideal weight.

The moral of the story? Cut snacking some slack!

It's not your enemy. In fact, if you do it right, it can actually be a huge help on your diet journey!

SUCCESS LESSON 22:

Your Four Quadrants

When it comes to your overall health, it's important to remember your life is really divided up into four main quadrants:

Mental	Emotional
Spiritual	Physical

One of the most interesting aspects of our lives is the fact that all of these areas are interconnected.

That means that when one area is off, the other areas are out of sync as well.

For example, have you ever noticed that when you catch a cold it's harder to feel mentally sharp?

Or, when you're going through a breakup you may feel physically drained as well?

That's one of the reasons why this book is designed the way it is.

You see, most diet programs will give you tips on how to improve your physical health—which is obviously a good place to start.

However, those programs fail to address the other three-fourths of your life!

My hope is that by including lessons that address the other quadrants of your life, you'll find this book will not only help you lose weight, but to truly be happier and healthier- for life!

You see, a program that only addresses your physical quadrant doesn't prepare you for the emotional challenges life throws at you. Nor does it help you think through how to reprogram your brain to work with you, instead of against you when you're trying to change. It also won't give you any insight on how to improve the spiritual aspect of your life.

Now, before I offend anyone, please know that I'm not going to espouse any religious viewpoints here. I simply mean that there's more to who we are than our body, thoughts, and feelings.

*In fact, the spiritual side of who we are may impact the world around us more than any of the others.

Have you ever known anyone who seems to carry a spirit of calmness? No matter what life throws at them, they seem to have an uncanny inner peace.

Or maybe you know someone who radiates joy everywhere they go? You can't spend time with them without walking away with a smile on your face.

These spiritual expressions are a result of being healthy in all four quadrants.

Why don't we see them in *everyone*?

In one respect, we do.

You see, even people who radiate negativity are spiritual. They're simply passing on the fruit of their ill-health (be it mental, emotional, or physical).

*The real question is, how is *your* spiritual health? What do you radiate to the people around you?

- Compassion or apathy?
- Kindness or cruelty?
- Understanding or indifference?

It's my belief that when we're *truly* healthy, our lives will emanate positivity as we become the best possible versions of ourselves.

Sound too new-agey?

Give it a little more thought, and I think you'll agree that there's something to all of this.

In fact, think back through the seasons of your life when you were at your happiest.

Were they the times when you were dealing with illness, or stress, or damaged relationships?

Or were they the times when you felt great, you were in a good mood, and your relationships were flourishing?

Like I said, I believe our four quadrants are all interconnected. And, whether you fully agree or not, just know that my hope is that this book will help to boost your health in any area where it might be lacking so you can truly experience life to its fullest.

What does "life to its fullest" look like?

You've already painted that picture for yourself: It's your Why!

Now, let's see what else we can do to bring that future to life!

LESSON 23:

Why Hunger Can Be A Good Thing

First, let me clarify that statement.

When I say "hunger," I'm not talking about extreme hunger or starvation. I'm talking about when you or I feel a little rumble in our belly that reminds us we haven't eaten for a while.

Why is this a good thing?

For years, many of us have been in the habit of eating because it's "lunch *time*" or "dinner *time*." The time on the Clock has had more to do with our eating habits than whether or not we were *actually* hungry.

This can be just as harmful as eating because we're bored or because we still have food left on our plate, even though we're already full.

This is where eating becomes just another form of entertainment. If we're not careful, it even opens the door to self-indulgence.

Am I suggesting that everything we eat has to be flavorless and our only concern should be nutritional value? Not at all.

I'm just challenging you to take a close look at the eating habits that got you where you are today.

I think you'll find, as I have, that eating for entertainment, eating because "it's time," and eating to clear our plate are all traps we've fallen into in the past.

What can we do to avoid these traps?

First, pick your foods based on their nutritional value, not their visual appeal.

Many fattening foods have fantastic flavors, but they also keep us from reaching our goals. Instead, look for ways to add flavor to healthy dishes served in healthy portions.

Second, be careful of eating simply because of the time on the clock.

I understand you may have to eat because it's your lunch break and you won't get another chance for four hours, and that's fine.

But when you have the option of eating at a certain time or waiting until you're actually hungry, try to wait for the actual hunger. It's your body's way of telling you it needs more fuel.

*Also, you have permission to never clear your plate again!

As I mentioned much earlier in the book, sometimes the best thing you can do is split a meal in half and take the leftovers with you. But there's also a freedom in eating part of your meal - to the point where you know you've had enough - and then pushing your plate away and calling it good.

It's actually kind of empowering. Try it sometime!

SUCCESS LESSON 23:

Accept No Substitutes

H ave you ever been misled by clever marketing?

You thought you were getting one thing, but you ended up getting something different instead.

In the restaurant world, in might come in the form of a burger that looks amazing in a picture, but then tastes like the person who prepared it was petting a wet dog and forgot to wash their hands. Plus, the burgers in the pictures are *always* bigger!

Or maybe you went to a movie after watching an exciting trailer only to find out that the only parts worth watching were in that same trailer, and the only exhilarating moment you experienced was when you almost lost your shoe to the sticky floor!

I had an experience like this when I was a teenager. My mom, my sister, and I were in California visiting family and decided to go to Hollywood. We parked and headed up to the strip to look at the famous handprints in the sidewalk. As we got close, a man skateboarded across the street in front of us and then puked all over a payphone.

Now, some people would say we parked in the wrong place.

Others would say that experience pretty much showed us the *real* Hollywood. The point is, we definitely didn't get what we were expecting...

Do you ever feel like you're living a *substitute life*?

You grew up expecting to find a clear path to your dreams, but then life happened, and you wound up far from where you thought you'd be.

I think this happens to many of us.

We wanted to be wealthy, successful, and attractive. We wanted an extravagant lifestyle, a picture-perfect family, and our dream job. We wanted to wake up every morning loving life and living our dreams.

Instead, our lives end up as pale reflections of the bold and beautiful visions we had for our future (if there's any resemblance whatsoever...)

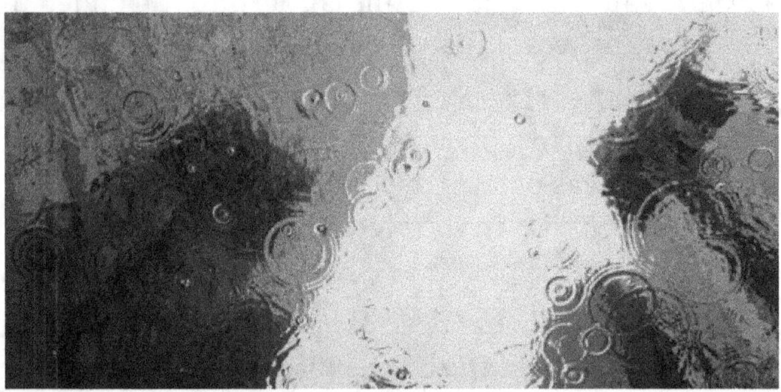

Now, you're probably wondering: Am I trying to stir up discontent in you?

No, and yes.

No, I don't want you to be unhappy with your life. I don't want you to dwell on how far away your reality is from the life of your dreams. And I don't want you to feel disappointed if you haven't achieved all of your goals in life.

However, I *do* want you to think about whether you've settled for a life that's a shadow of the one you dreamed of.

I get it. Life throws curve balls at all of us.

- We face challenges we never expected.
- We make choices we regret.
- We make sacrifices for people we care about.
- We get sidetracked by good things and let go of our big dreams.

As some people would say, "Reality sets in…"

*But what if the life of your dreams is the life you were *meant* to live?

What if you could still have the future you longed for as a child?

I believe we know ourselves much better as children than we do as adults. Somewhere along the way, our dreams get buried under the expectations of others, and we lose sight of them. Or we hit enough walls that we simply give up on them.

We settle.

Isn't that what happened to most of us?

We gave up. We lost hope. We surrendered.

And yet, *how many of us would tell our children to do that?*

How many parents have you heard say, "Now, don't dream *too* big!" Or "Oh, you'll never be a millionaire. Maybe you should just set your sights on being a gas station attendant instead." (No offense, gas station attendants).

Here's my point: As you continue working towards your Why and achieving your weight-loss goals, why not revive some of the other goals you've had for your life?

If you're going to change your *body* for the better, why not change the other things in your life that you're not satisfied with?

- Why not look for a better job?
- Why not get more education too?

- And why not dare to dream again?

We look at the lives of people we admire, and we think "I wish I could have what *they* have."

The truth is, you have that same potential within *you*!

Is this true for every circumstance? No.

Having a figure skater build will make it hard to become an NFL linebacker.

But if some part of you longs for a better life, don't stifle that longing. Pursue it!

As Jim Rohn said, "For things to change, *you* have to change. Don't wish it was easier, wish you were better. Don't wish for less problems, wish for more skills. Don't wish for less challenge, wish for more wisdom."

Don't settle for a substitute life.

Instead, go for the life you *really* want. Even if you don't get everything you dreamt of as a child, at least no one can accuse you of giving up.

So, for now, let's keep going until we get you to your weight-loss goals. But after that, I dare you to see what other dreams you can accomplish!

LESSON 24:

Learn to Savor Every Bite

Think about how fortunate we are for just a moment.

For most of us, there's food waiting in the fridge whenever we want it. We have money to go out and buy more when our pantry's empty. And most of us haven't ever had to know what it's like to be desperately hungry.

Millions of people on our planet are living a very different story. They're constantly hungry, and their days are spent doing whatever they can to find their next meal.

Am I saying that to make you feel guilty? No.

I'm saying this to remind all of us of the *importance of gratitude*.

When we lose perspective on how fortunate we are to have our next meal readily available and we begin to take food for granted, we can become self-indulgent.

I'm not saying this from up on my high horse, I'm saying it because I'm more guilty than many people of shoveling food down my throat without ever taking a second to taste what I'm eating.

I take it for granted, instead of being grateful for what I have and savoring each bite.

Let's decide today to be different.

As we discussed before, how many times do we gather around a table with our family and friends and spend the meal with our attention focused on our *food* instead of the *people* sitting around us?

We eat dinner at the same table but we're not *really* together. We're not connecting.

Food can become an idol that we worship.

I can tell you that I didn't get to be over 70 pounds overweight by keeping food in its proper place.

Slow down.

Appreciate each bite.

But more than that, appreciate the people who are gathered around the table with you.

*Unplug yourself and your kids from your phones and spend some quality time together.

It makes me so sad to see families out to eat "together," but they couldn't be farther apart. They aren't talking, they aren't engaged, they aren't really present.

Let's change this.

Let's start putting aside distractions and really being together at mealtimes.

I love the stories of families shutting off their phones and setting them aside at dinner.

I love to see happy families laughing and having a good time around the table.

They've learned to savor life one bite at a time.

Let's do the same thing!

SUCCESS LESSON 24:

How is Your Inner Life?

As I mentioned before, one of the things that makes this book different is its emphasis on improving your inner life, even while we're working on improving your outer life. I believe this two-fold approach to diet success is what's made the biggest difference for me in terms of losing weight and keeping it off.

*What good is a diet that helps you shed all your unwanted weight, but doesn't also show you a better way to live?

As soon as you're done with the diet, all your old habits will come flooding back in, because it hasn't helped you to live a happier, healthier *inner* life.

It's like driving through a car wash, but then bypassing the vacuum. Sure, the outside looks great, but the inside's still a mess!

Dale Carnegie's How to Stop Worrying and Start Living is a timeless book that addresses this subject from many angles. In the book, he quotes Marcus Aurelius as saying, *"Our life is what our thoughts make it."*

Carnegie goes on to say, "Yes, if we think happy thoughts, we will be happy. If we think miserable thoughts, we will be miserable. If we think fear thoughts, we will be fearful. If we think sickly thoughts, we will probably be ill. If we think failure, we will certainly fail."

What have *you* been thinking?

As I mentioned before, depression has been a serious struggle for me on my journey. I've allowed it to lead me into all sorts of unhealthy thoughts and habits. And it all happened because of an unhealthy inner life.

Remember our discussion of the power of "what if?" It can be our greatest ally, or our fiercest enemy.

The darkest seasons of my life have been flooded with cycles of negative "what ifs." Maybe it's been the same for you.

We start to turn all of our worries into "what ifs."

- What if I get sick?
- What if I get fired?
- What if they reject me?
- What if I fail?

In the midst of all of these worries, we become paralyzed.

How could we *not*? Every ounce of our mental energy is focused on why our efforts *won't* work. We're expecting the worst, and we often get what we expect.

Fortunately, because of the power of our thoughts in our life, we can turn our attitude (and our entire life) around with positive what ifs!

- What if I stay healthy into my 80's? How much could I accomplish?!
- What if I get a promotion? What would I do if I got a significant raise?
- What if they love me? Who knows what kind of future we could have together?!
- What if I succeed? If I can achieve *this* goal, who knows what else I could do?!

Are you starting to see the power of *transforming your thought life?*

Practice it right now!

Write out your five biggest worries in "what if" question form. What are the things that are keeping you up at night?

Once you put them down on paper, write out their hopeful opposites. (Like I did above).

Here's an example:

"What if I go through this program and I don't lose any weight?" turns into "What if I go through this program and I achieve my weight-loss goal? What *other* goal could I start to pursue next?"

In effect, what we're doing is reprogramming our negative thought cycle and turning it into a positive/hopeful thought cycle.

*Instead of staring at our problems, we're looking for possibilities.

In this way, by transforming our thoughts, we begin to transform our life (inside *and* out!)

LESSON 25:

Give Up Eating for Entertainment

Your taste buds are like needy little kids. They want constant attention and stimulation. They want to be entertained and spoiled with sweets and new and exciting flavors.

It's time to start denying your taste buds.

Part of finding success in your diet is learning to stop eating for entertainment; and, instead, start eating food for its nutritional value.

Now, I love tasty food as much as the next person.

I spent years indulging my appetite and packing on the pounds as I made one unhealthy dietary choice after another. Washing calories down with more calories—and all of it tasted great!

But then I saw where all of those empty calories had taken me.

- 70 pounds overweight.
- Lethargic and lazy.
- Depressed and disheartened.

Was it worth it? Heck no!

Was there a quick and easy Reset button? Nope.

I had to start working the pounds off one at a time, just like I put them on.

So, what are some strategies to start turning this around?

- <u>Pay attention to the "lack of nutrition" facts</u>- A lot of the time, if we'll take a second to look at the calorie count on a dessert, it becomes much easier to turn it down.

  The same goes for fast food meals. If you're doing well at keeping your calories down and the number five combo weighs in at 900 to 1500 calories, it's time to move on.

  No one meal or dessert is worth *that* many calories when you're trying to lose weight.

- <u>Substitute healthy sweets for fattening sweets</u>- Cravings happen. So do sweet tooths (sweet teeth?)…

  Don't be afraid of them, and don't give in to them. Plan for them.

  Have healthy snacks on hand for when these cravings occur. It might be a pack of organic fruit snacks or a piece of fresh fruit or a couple of cans of fruit set aside for a fruit salad.

  Whatever works for you is fine. Just be ready.

You'll end up finding out the most amazing things:

- You *can* pass on dessert.
- You can forego that amazing new burger or sandwich.
- You can live without whatever new dish your eyes and taste buds so desire.

The cravings will pass. And, on the other side, you'll emerge stronger and healthier for having passed on those treats and kept your eyes on your goal instead.

SUCCESS LESSON 25:

Letting Go of Distractions

What do you turn to in order to keep from dealing with the problems in your life?

You see, distractions are double-edged: Some are <u>in</u>vasive, others are <u>e</u>vasive.

Some distractions bombard us from the outside like pop-up ads.

The distractions I want to address here are the ones we choose to pursue in order to take our minds off of the issues we're facing in life.

In her book <u>The Gifts of Imperfection</u>, Brené Brown talks about the behaviors we turn to in order to numb emotions like vulnerability and shame.

She says, "We can anesthetize with a whole bunch of stuff, including alcohol, drugs, food, sex, relationships, money, work, caretaking, gambling, staying busy, affairs, chaos, shopping, planning, perfectionism, constant change, and the Internet."

If you're like me, *some of those things hit really close to home.*

For our purposes, let's focus on numbing with food.

As we saw earlier, sugar can be as addictive as any drug (if not *more* addictive). And food can become a coping mechanism for many of us along the way.

On a deeper level, we may actually turn to destructive eating habits out of a sense of self-loathing. We are, in effect, punishing ourselves with food.

"Why not?" we ask ourselves. "Nobody cares about me anyway."

For some of you, that sounds completely foreign. And that's a good thing.

However, if you're reading that, and it hits home, just know that you're not the only one who's felt that way. One of the worst aspects of depression is that we can turn our anger inwards and become self-destructive even at the level of our eating habits.

If your depression is at that level right now, know that there *is* hope. You *can* find your way back to a happier, healthier life. I know it's possible, because it's a part of *my* story.

Fortunately, it doesn't have to be the *end* of our story. In fact, just being here right now means that you have the opportunity to change everything in your life for the better!

Later in that same chapter, Brené says, "Whether we're overcoming adversity, surviving trauma, or dealing with stress and anxiety, having a sense of purpose, meaning, and perspective in our lives allows us to develop understanding and move forward."

How do you find your purpose? Look at your Why!

Pursuing that purpose has led you this far, and I believe it can carry you through the rest of this book and on to the point of reaching your ideal weight.

From there, you have to discover an even deeper sense of meaning in your life.

What were you put on this earth to do?

Personally, I find meaning in writing and encouraging people. I love the idea of helping people live happier, healthier lives. It fuels me with a passion I can hardly put into words!

What are you passionate about?

There are a couple ways to discover your passion.

1. <u>What makes you come alive?</u> What do you do that lights a spark of energy and enthusiasm within you? It could be singing, writing, helping people, giving, or any number of things.

2. <u>What makes you angry?</u> What injustice in the world really sets you off? Your passion may lie in fighting to eliminate this issue from the world, whether that's poverty, hunger, homelessness, abuse, or some other cultural malady.

Howard Thurman has been quoted as saying, "Don't ask yourself what the world needs. Ask yourself what makes you come alive, and go do that, because what the world needs is people who have come alive."

I would encourage you to look at your purpose from both perspectives:

What does the world need from you that only *you* can contribute?

What do you love to do that makes you come alive?

Somewhere within the answers to those two questions lies a passion worth giving your life to.

I hope you'll find it and live it out.

The world is waiting!

Be sure to take some time and explore this topic out loud with a friend or family member. Ask them what they're passionate about, and then look for ways to put your passions into action!

LESSON 26:

Avoiding HALTS in Your Diet

In the recovery movement, one of the things they teach is that we tend to make our worst decisions when we are Hungry, Angry, Lonely, Tired, or Stressed. Hence the acronym HALTS.

Does this resonate with your story?

Have you ever been Hungry and grabbed something quick to eat, only to regret it later?

Have you ever been Angry and said or done something you wound up apologizing for later?

Have you ever been so Lonely that you resorted to hanging out with someone you didn't even really like?

Have you ever been so Tired that you had trouble thinking straight?

Have you ever been so Stressed out that you made an impulsive decision, only to regret it moments later?

How do we deal with these threats to our diet success?

- <u>Hunger</u>- Do your best to make sure you're never extremely hungry. Like we talked about before, a little hunger is actually a good thing, it lets you know that your body needs more fuel.

Be sure to keep healthy snack foods on hand, so you can eat something that's good for you if your appetite flares up.

- <u>Anger</u>- This is a tough one. No matter how hard we try, it seems like there are always things that get under our skin.

  It could be other people's words or actions. It might also come as the result of our own mistakes.

  One thing I find helpful when I'm angry is pausing before I react to make sure I don't say or do something I'll regret.

*I also stop and think about things I'm grateful for. It's almost impossible to be grateful and angry at the same time.

- <u>Lonely</u>- I'm a firm believer that the wrong kind of company can be worse than being alone. So be careful who you reach out to.

  With that being said, make sure that you *do* reach out when you're feeling lonely.

  It helps to have friends and family who've given you permission to reach out to them at any time.

  Sometimes just getting out and being around people (in the right context) can help too. However, be careful that you don't ever make food your companion. It will let you down every time. And it's a terrible conversationalist...

- <u>Tired</u>- We're not at our best when we're exhausted. Our immune system is weaker. Our endurance is lower. And we often make poor choices.

  If you're living a lifestyle that runs you ragged, consider making changes that will slow down the pace of life for you.

Many of our worst meal choices come when we're "on the go."

- <u>Stressed</u>- We can do some pretty dumb things when we're stressed out. Often, we reach out for anything we think might numb the pain and lower our stress level.

As we discussed recently, one of the coping mechanisms many of us turn to is food.

Why? Because it's considered by many people to be a lesser evil. But in the end, it can still have serious consequences.

And it doesn't do anything to fix the problem that stressed us out to begin with!

The only way to stop stress is to address the stressor directly—whether that's a person or a situation.

So, there you have them. The five biggest obstacles to your diet success.

Now that we've identified them, the question is, what will you *do* about them?

I recommend going through the list again and looking at how these hindrances have been showing up in your life. Be super-specific as you identify them.

- When are you most susceptible to hunger?
- What situations tend to make you angry?
- When are you at your loneliest?
- What activities in your life leave you feeling tired?
- What are the issues in your life that are stressing you out?

Once you identify these things, you can start to change them. If you can't change the situation itself, you can still change how you respond to it.

If you feel like your life is out of control and you're powerless to influence the things that are causing the HALTS in your life, it's time for you to develop healthy self-interest.

I'm not encouraging you to only think about yourself (that's *selfishness*).

Self-interest simply means you think about yourself the same way you would anyone else.

- You cut yourself some slack.
- You give yourself grace when you mess up.
- You take time to take care of yourself.

When you develop a sense of healthy self-interest, not only will you begin to get your HALTS under control, you'll also begin to enjoy life more. And you'll be a more enjoyable person to be around!

You'll be amazed at who you become when you let go of perfectionism, accept the fact that you're just as human as anyone else, and there's nothing wrong with that!

And if the HALTS ever start to feel overwhelming, you can always ask a friend for help. (More on *that* subject soon…)

SUCCESS LESSON 26:

Living a Life of Integrity

There's a model I developed several years ago that I want to share with you now. It helps us see how we became the person we are today; which, in turn, can give us some ideas about how to change and become the person we want to be.

The model is called: Identity Reintegration Theory.

Let's take a look at each of the stages:
- Integration- From the moment we're born, we begin taking in information. Everything we see, hear, smell, taste, touch, and feel is processed on one level or another. We develop our early beliefs about people and the world, as well as many of our early habits during this time.

- Disintegration- When we hit adolescence, our world starts to fall apart. We realize that we have a choice in who we become. We begin to struggle with our identity and experiment to find out who we really want to be.

- Reintegration- As we enter young adulthood, the pieces start to come back together. We begin to make decisions about who we are, what we believe, and what we value.

- <u>Further Identity Formation</u>- In our early adulthood, most of us are still open to the possibility of change. This is especially true of people with families, as they have to grow and adapt to support their spouse and children in an ever-changing world.

- <u>Identity Fixation</u>- At some point in our lives, we become much less malleable. We decide that we've gone as far as we're going to go, and we're done changing. Our personalities become fixed to a large degree. At this point, we either wind up as a person of integrity, living a fulfilled life; or we suffer from a lack of integrity, and feel like our life is incomplete.

What's the point of this model?

It shows how we develop over time. It shows the stages when we're most open to change and how we became the people we are today.

For most of us, the habits and behaviors that have shaped us came along sometime during our early lives, and we simply incorporated them into our identity.

We looked at potential defining behaviors and decided whether or not we wanted them to be a part of who we were becoming.

These decisions influenced our diet, our habits, our relationships, our careers, our personalities, and every other aspect of our lives.

Who we are today is either based on a sense of integrity and self-assurance, or it's based on a lack of integrity and self-doubt.

Which option better describes *you*?

Do you feel like you're living a fulfilled life, or do you feel like something's missing?

There is a certain beauty to living a life of contentment.

I don't mean that we settle for where we are and stop striving to better ourselves. I just mean that we're happy with who we are (inside and out) and we're no longer chasing after the acceptance and approval of other people.

*Now, here's the good news: If you're unhappy with where you're at in life, you don't have to stay there!

Can it be harder to change later in life? Definitely.

Is it ever *impossible* to change? No way!

Here's my three-part challenge to you:

1. Take a moment to picture your funeral. Who's there? What are they saying about you? Write those things down.
2. Next, write down what you *want* people to say about you. How do you hope people will remember you when you're gone?
3. Write down the changes you would need to make between now and the end of your life in order to become *that* person.

Here's an example:

1. People would say that I had a gift for writing, but I never really did anything with it.
2. I want people to say that I lived life to the fullest and achieved my dream of becoming a published author.
3. I'm going to do everything I can between now and then to bring my dream of becoming a writer to life!

Go back to the seven areas of goal setting we talked about before:

1. Financial Goals
2. Career/Business Goals
3. Free Time/Family Time Goals
4. Health/Appearance Goals

5. Relationship Goals
6. Personal Growth Goals
7. Making A Difference/Legacy Goals

What would you like people to say about each of these areas of your life?

If you're not satisfied with your life in one or more areas, what changes do you need to make?

Now, *what's one step you can take today to move toward becoming the person you'd like to be at the end of your life?*

From there, map out the other changes you'd like to make. Then start setting goals and working toward them until the person you see in the mirror each day slowly becomes the person you want your family and friends to remember when you're gone.

Will making these changes be a huge challenge for many of us? Sure, but what do you have to lose?

Set your goal on becoming the person you were born to be (the best possible version of yourself). Then set out to become that person because of what it will make of you to achieve it!

You never know where you might end up, or who you could end up inspiring on your journey!

LESSON 27:

When you embark on your diet journey, be sure to recruit your friends and family.

Let them know what you're doing, and make sure they also know your Why.

It might sound like this: "I wanted to let you know that I'm starting on a plant-based diet. I want to lose weight and be happier and healthier so I can <u>(insert your Why)</u>."

- Play with my kids/grandkids.
- Feel better about myself.
- Get back the self-confidence I lost when I started gaining weight.
- Look and feel great again.

Whatever your reason is, put it out there for the world to see. This will help them support you in your goals. And most of them will also be careful to avoid tempting you with foods that would throw off your diet and keep you from reaching your goal.

The really good ones will be there to listen when you call them and say: "Hey, I really want to order and eat an entire Canadian bacon pizza, so I need you to distract me!"

They'll also help you when it comes to eating out and you're thinking about ordering something that'll interfere with your diet.

If you try to order a burger and a Coke, they'll tell you to order a salad and a water instead.

Friends and family members like this are priceless! They're the ones who will help you keep going when the going gets tough.

The key to good accountability is asking for it, so be sure to take that step. Whether it's with a parent, spouse, child, or friend, let them know specifically what you're trying to accomplish and why.

*Ask them to say something if they see you slipping into old habits.

It might even annoy you sometimes, but what won't annoy you is seeing your weight drop five pounds after a week of healthy eating. Instead, you'll be jazzed to see if you can do it again the next week!

You could also invite your accountability partner(s) to join you on your diet journey. They could become your exercise buddy and *literally* be there with you every step of the way.

Ultimately, it helps to have cheerleaders. People who will support you in reaching your goal.

This may also mean putting more distance between yourself and the people who would hinder you in your progress by encouraging you to pick up old bad habits.

One last suggestion: Once you find your accountability partner (or partners) give them a specific list of questions to ask you.

These might be questions like:

- Did you get your two miles in today?
- Are you staying away from sugar?
- Are you sticking to your plan?
- Where do you feel like you're struggling?

- Is there anything I can do to better support you?

With this kind of accountability and support, you will springboard yourself toward success in reaching your weight-loss goals.

Plus, your success may be the thing that inspires your friends, family members, or coworkers to go after their own dreams and goals!

SUCCESS LESSON 27:

Who Could You Inspire?

I want to stay with this subject for a little while, because I believe some of you are probably already dismissing the idea from that last sentence.

"*I* could never inspire anyone..." you're telling yourself. But you're wrong!

You have no idea who in your life might be looking up to you on a daily basis.

- Your kids.
- Your significant other.
- Your friends.
- Your coworkers.
- People you meet in passing.

*There's no telling how many people could benefit from seeing you lead a happier, healthier life!

Think about it this way, we all have people we try to steer clear of at work, right?

We run because we know that, if we don't, we'll end up getting stuck listening to all the things that are going wrong in that person's life... These people can *literally* suck the energy right out of you.

However, you also probably know people who are the opposite of the energy suckers.

These are the people who live inspiring lives.

No, they're not necessarily heroes we worship. They're just the kind of people who leave us feeling better after we encounter them.

These people tend to be positive most of the time. They're upbeat and proactive. They're the kind of person we turn to when we need advice.

And, believe it or not, *you* can be one of these people.

In fact, I can guarantee some of you already are.

For others of us, it may take a little bit of intentionality to become this type of person, but I honestly believe anyone can inspire others.

Think about the people you've looked up to the most in your life. Maybe it was a teacher, an employer, a pastor, or a friend. What made you look up to them?

- Did they see the best in everyone they met?
- Did they take time to *really* listen to you?
- Did they tend to look on the bright side in any situation?
- Were they compassionate and encouraging?
- Did spending time with them make you want to be a better person?

Having these people in our lives is a gift.

Fortunately, I come from a family full of these people!

Here's my point: Inside of you, there's an inspiring person waiting to break free!

You have everything you need inside of you to become the kind of person who breathes new life into the lives of the people around them.

Think back to the people who've inspired you. What would you say defined them?

- Love, joy, patience, kindness, forgiveness, empathy, enthusiasm?

None of these things are genetic traits. They're intentional ways of living that anyone can put into action.

And, when we begin living out these virtues on a regular basis, they become more and more natural over time.

So, what's the best way to begin practicing these attributes (or any others you might come up with)?

Benjamin Franklin chose 13 such virtues and focused on one per week.

I recommend making a list of seven and then choosing one to focus on each day.

How much different would your life be if you sought to live out one of these attributes from the time you woke up to the time you went to bed every day?

- How would it affect your family?
- How would it affect your coworkers?
- How would it affect people who don't even know you?

You see, we tend to underestimate the impact we can have on the world around us.

We think, "I could never be as inspiring as So and So…" But it's just not true.

The problem is that when we think of changing the world, we think it requires a grand achievement like solving world hunger.

The fact is, one small act of kindness can create a ripple effect that could literally make a difference in thousands of lives.

In this way, by changing *your* world, you're actually changing *the* world!

Here's my challenge to you: Pick a list of virtues you want to live out.

If you're having trouble coming up with seven of them, think back to the exercise we did on how we want people to remember us at our funeral. Pick the seven traits you most want to be remembered for, then start focusing on one each day.

You can write it on a note card and carry it in your pocket or set up a reminder in your phone every morning.

The important thing is to look for opportunities to put these attributes into practice *every day*!

If we'll do this, before long we'll become just like those inspiring people we talked about before.

And, in the end, our world will be a happier, healthier place too!

LESSON 28:

*A Little More on Recruiting
Your Friends*

First, please know this isn't about selling more books. It's about making sure you have all the support you can get.

Losing weight isn't easy. If it was, everyone would be doing it!

What makes the difference for many people is knowing they're not alone.

Now, I can and will remind you of that from my side of things as much as possible, but I can't be there for you like the people you see every day can.

I can't get up and go for a walk with you or hop onto the treadmill beside you, but your good friends can. So, be sure to seriously consider asking them to join you.

Want to know a great time to ask? When you've started to shed a few pounds, and your friend notices, it's a great time to invite them to join you!

They might say something like: "Wow, that diet's really working for you!" Or "Have you lost some weight?"

Let them know that you have, and you'd love for them to join you.

Here's the deal: Eating right and exercising is easy on the days when you're making regular progress. It's harder when you plateau for a while and you have to push to break through and get those next few pounds off.

Knowing your accountability partner is going to be there waiting for you that next day can make all the difference at times like these!

You'll also get the benefit of being able to encourage them in *their* journey! Plus, you can help them keep going if they need some inspiration along the way.

You can be like a coach to them in their tough times, and you'll also get to celebrate with them as they hit their milestones!

Other fun ways to bring your friends along for the ride are things like taste testing. "Hey, I found a new recipe for a vegan lasagna."

Or shopping for smaller clothes. "Hey, so all my pants are two sizes too big now, will you come shopping with me?"

These types of activities will keep you working together and encouraging each other.

They're also great ways for your friend to see where they could be if they keep going on their own diet.

Plus, being a role model or mentor is a great way to keep yourself disciplined on your own journey.

Do you have an accountability partner in mind?

If so, be sure to reach out to them today!

SUCCESS LESSON 28:

Doing the Impossible

"**I**t's time to stop letting your history control your destiny."

This is one of my favorite lines from Andy Andrews' book <u>The Noticer</u>. If you haven't read it, be sure to pick it up sometime.

That line comes up during a conversation about worry. And, in this lesson, I want to talk about a subject that can trigger worry in the best of us: Change.

When you think of change, what words come to mind?

Do you think: fun, adventure, and excitement?

Or do you think: scary, different, and difficult?

Many people believe *change is impossible.*

For a lot of us, change is one of the scariest things in life. We'd rather stay in predictable misery than risk changing.

And we do.

- We stay in jobs we loathe.
- We stay in relationships we hate.
- We stay addicted.
- We stay overweight.
- We stay stuck.

Because living with all of these things is easier than risking change.

I still remember my Crisis Counseling professor in college saying, "Any major change in life brings about a crisis."

Having lived a lot more life since then, I have to agree.

And yet, that statement also raises an important question: What if it's worth going through the crisis to reach a better place in life?

I'll be the first to admit, I've struggled with a change phobia most of my life. I prefer predictability and routine. I love consistency.

But, like many people, I became a slave to these things and found myself living an unhappy and unhealthy life.

Can you relate?

I mean, change is *hard*, isn't it? It's a struggle.

And that leads me to one of the best quotes I've ever come across: "Every true strength is gained through struggle."

Here's my point: If you've made it this far in this book, you're a stronger person than you were when you began it.

- You've faced your fear of the unknown, and you've kept going.
- You've made lifestyle choices many people aren't brave enough to make.
- You've persevered in your journey to find a happier, healthier life.
- You've made up your mind not to let your history control your destiny, and that's an amazing feat!

And so, since you've come this far, keep going!

We only have a couple more lessons left to cover together (though you're welcome to read back through them as often as you'd like).

With that in mind, my hope is that, as we've been on this journey together, you've seen yourself grow as a person even as you've begun to lose your unwanted weight.

In the end, if I only help you shed a few pounds along the way, that's okay. But my hope is that, even as your plant-based diet helps you get closer to your ideal weight, you're also discovering (or re-discovering) your inner strength and your incredible potential!

You see, I believe if you can summon up the strength to work through this book and reach your ideal weight, there's no limit to what you can accomplish!

Far too many people "lead lives of quiet desperation" (as Thoreau said). They stay in their unhealthy habits and routines until their bodies break down, or *even worse*, until their spirits are broken.

*But that's not *your* story!

You've decided to look change in the eye and keep on going! And it's my sincere hope that, as you've been scaling this brick wall, you've begun to understand that there's no wall you can't scale and no dream in your heart you can't realize!

As we move on and knock out these last couple lessons, don't ever overlook the courage and strength it's taken you to come this far.

You're doing the impossible, and you're doing great!

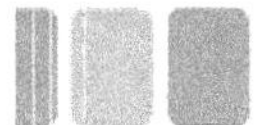 # Plant-Based Diet Success
Success Accelerators

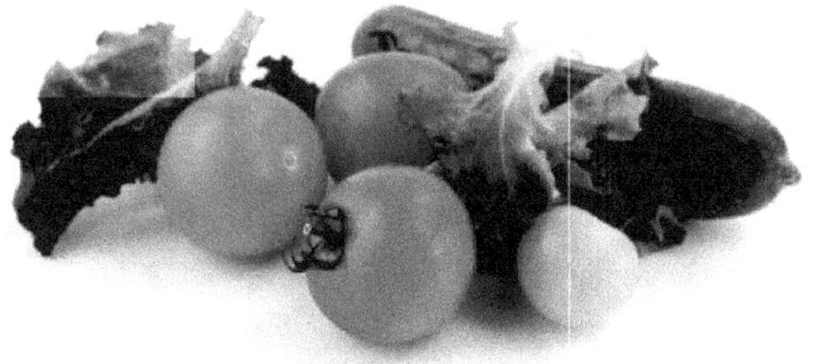

LESSON 29:

Maintaining Your Progress

"**W**hat do I do once I reach my ideal weight?"

This is a step many diet programs skip.

You get the weight off, and then you celebrate! Woo Hoo!

- You go out and guzzle down that milkshake you've been craving.
- You scarf down the steak you've been denying yourself.
- And you slurp a sugary soft drink to wash it down.

This is what you've been working towards, right?

Here's the deal: That is absolutely one way you can go.

You can get all of the weight off and go back to your old way of eating. All your favorite foods are there waiting for you!

I wouldn't recommend that. But it's certainly an option.

Instead of potentially throwing away all your hard work and gaining back the weight you lost, I would encourage you to adopt a different plan.

Consider coming up with a plan that lets you enjoy some of your old favorites, without risking all the progress you've made.

The truth is, I've made great strides in losing weight in the past, only to gain it all back. But with the plant-based diet, I found a way to drop the pounds *and keep them off*.

That's what I want for you.

Here's how I'm doing it:

First, figure out your ideal weight window. It's the window of around 10 pounds where you find that you feel your best. For me, this is between 160 and 170 pounds.

Next, find a balance which allows you to eat some of your favorite foods, without going back to all of your old eating habits. I recommend starting with one meal a week where you eat one of your old favorites. Keep the rest of your meals plant-based for the time being.

Now, the key is to pay careful attention to how you feel and how your body processes this food. If you feel sluggish or nauseated, it may be best to stick with the plan that's been working for you. If not, you may be okay to enjoy a couple of meat meals in a week.

From here, you can scale things up accordingly. You may be able to reintroduce meat and dairy products into all of your meals, or it may be better to keep at least two of your daily meals plant-based.

In the end, if you start gaining some weight back, you can always switch back to the plant-based diet until you're back within your weight window. It's just like adjusting a thermostat!

Super simple, right?

SUCCESS LESSON 29:

Living "As If"

In this lesson, I want to share another lesson drawn from one of Jack Canfield's Success Principles with you. Principle 12 is simply titled "Act As If."

As Jack says, "Once you choose what it is you want to be, do, or have… the proper order of things is to start now and *be* who you want to be, then *do* the actions that go along with being that person, and soon you will find that you easily *have* everything you want in life—health, wealth, fulfilling relationships, and social impact."

There's a good chance you haven't reached your ideal weight yet. And that's okay! As we discussed before, weight loss is a process, not an overnight change.

However, since you've come this far, now's a great time to begin acting as if you've already reached your weight-loss goal.

What will this do for you?

- It will immediately transform your self-confidence.
- It will change how you eat (especially in terms of portion sizes).
- It will guide your decisions from this point forward.

Before every decision you make, ask yourself, "Is this what the *old* me would've done, or is this what the *new* me would do?"

Then go with the new. Every time.

From this point forward, the choices you make will inevitably lead you to where you want to go, in every area of your life.

It's like the GPS we talked about earlier.

You know what to do because you know where you're going. You have a set destination, and *nothing's* going to get in your way.

When you have that kind of resolve, you have everything you need to bring your dream to life.

So, take another moment to picture the future you've dreamed of. Think about what it would look like for you to achieve your goals in every area of your life.

Hold that image in your heart and mind. Let it sink in until you feel it in every part of your being.

Then, once you truly believe the potential to become that person is already inside you, all you have to do is make one choice after another in line with that vision. And, sooner or later, you'll get there.

Now, go live as the person who can make all of your dreams a reality!

LESSON 30:

The New You! Success!

If you follow the plan I've laid out for you, I truly believe the day will come when you'll reach your ideal weight.

If you're there now, that's awesome! Congratulations!

If you're still working on it, congratulations! Your dedication and discipline are successes in and of themselves. Keep going, and you *will* reach your goal.

So, what do you do when you reach your ideal weight?

My first suggestion is to celebrate by embracing your Why—whatever it was.

If it was playing with your kids or grandkids, take them out to the park and fly a kite or run around or play catch.

These are simple and beautiful ways to bask in your success and share it with the people who matter most to you.

If your Why was to lose weight and look great, go out with a friend and buy some of the clothes you always wanted, but couldn't fit into.

If you were like me, you've probably dropped a size or two (or more). Celebrate by buying some clothes that accent your new figure. You might even ask your friend to take some pictures you can send to family and friends who've been cheering you on.

Does that sound kind of vain? It isn't! You've worked your butt off (literally!) to get here. Take the time to recognize that and enjoy your feeling of success.

You've done what millions of people only dream of doing, and what you yourself might have believed was impossible before starting this diet.

You are a champion! Don't ever sell yourself short or underestimate the magnitude of what you've accomplished.

"But anyone could do this…" you might say. And there's some truth to that statement. *But most people won't.* That's what makes *you* so special!

You took action where others wouldn't. You did the hard work others won't.

Now you get to live the life you've dreamed of and enjoy the results of your efforts. And that's something you can and should be proud of.

Rest assured that I'm proud of you!

This book (and the lessons in it) is my effort to pay it forward to others who are facing the same struggles I faced, and I hope you'll do the same! Whether that's coming alongside someone you know who's on their own diet journey, or just directing them to plantbaseddietsuccess.com, either way is great!

Here's wishing you all the best in your new life!

SUCCESS LESSON 30:

Your Next Success

So, now that you've achieved weight-loss success, what area of your life will you focus on next?

- Financial success?
- Relationship success?
- Career success?

Your ability to follow through and reach your ideal weight tells me you can achieve success in *anything* you choose.

My advice: Dream big! After all, that's what got you here.

- You cast a vision for the life of your dreams.
- You believed in your vision every step of the way.
- You fueled that vision with passion and enthusiasm.
- And then you took action until you reached your goal!

You've followed Walt Disney's formula for success: *Dream, Believe, Dare, Do!*

If you can do that when it comes to weight loss, why couldn't you do it in any other area of your life?

You see, my hope is that this book has given you more than just a thinner body. Sure, I'm hoping you've been able to slim down to your ideal weight, but that's just the beginning!

What I *truly* want is for you to walk away from this book with increased self-confidence, renewed passion for life, and a burning desire to achieve your dreams for *every* area of your life!

That's what this book has *really* been about.

So, yes, you should absolutely celebrate your weight-loss success!

But don't let the journey end there.

Instead, pick up some of the resources I've suggested throughout this book. Let them fuel you with the same desire for success that led me to start Plant-Based Diet Success, and then go out and change your world!

Live a life that will inspire your family, your friends, and people you haven't even met yet!

That's my true hope for you: Not *just* a happier, healthier life, but an *inspired* and *fulfilled* life!

Here's the real danger you'll face as you walk away from this book: going back to living an unchanged, uninspired life.

You see, many of us tend to gloss over our successes. We minimize them. We tell ourselves, "Anyone could've done *that*." And we slip back into old habits and behaviors.

The label we put on ourselves says: Nothing Special.

*Don't *ever* do that to yourself again!

What you've done here *is* special! It *does* matter! It *is* significant!

In fact, it's the launching point for the life of your dreams! The foundation for an exceptional life!

So, take off!

- Dream even bigger dreams for yourself, and the people you love!
- Believe in your dreams, just like you believed you could reach your weight-loss goals!
- Dare to fuel your dreams with passion and enthusiasm!
- Do whatever it takes to bring those dreams to life, and

to help the people around you live the lives of *their* dreams as well!

You've opened the door to a new and inspiring life, now walk through it!

This brick wall is in the past, now it's time to take on the next one!

No matter what your life was like before this accomplishment, from this point on, know that you are astonishing!

Most of all, I want you to know that it has been an honor and a privilege for me to join you on this journey.

You truly are an inspiration to me, and to so many others!

Your life is a gift and a blessing! Thank you for sharing a part of it with me!

Now, get out there and change *your* world!

To your *continued* success!

Josh

ABOUT THE AUTHOR:

Josh is on a mission to help hundreds of thousands of people live happier, healthier lives!

From an early age, his family instilled in him a love of writing and a desire to help people reach their full potential. Being the son of two brilliant entrepreneurs who created an innovative aquaponics greenhouse system also gave him the gifts of outside-the-box thinking and dreaming big dreams!

Josh graduated from Ozark Christian College in Joplin, Missouri with a degree in Christian Ministry and Psychology and a desire to change the world. And even through the ups and downs of his life since that time, he's held onto his passion for encouraging people to pursue the life of their dreams!

In 2017, when Josh's weight had skyrocketed to 245 pounds, he knew he had to make some serious changes to get his life (and his health) back on track. By following a plant-based diet, he was able to surpass his initial weight-loss goals and lose 80 pounds! His diet success also reawakened his passion for helping other people live inspired lives.

This book was born from the lessons he discovered during the course of his journey.

To learn more about Josh's weight-loss journey and the benefits of a plant-based diet, check out his website: plantbaseddietsuccess.com

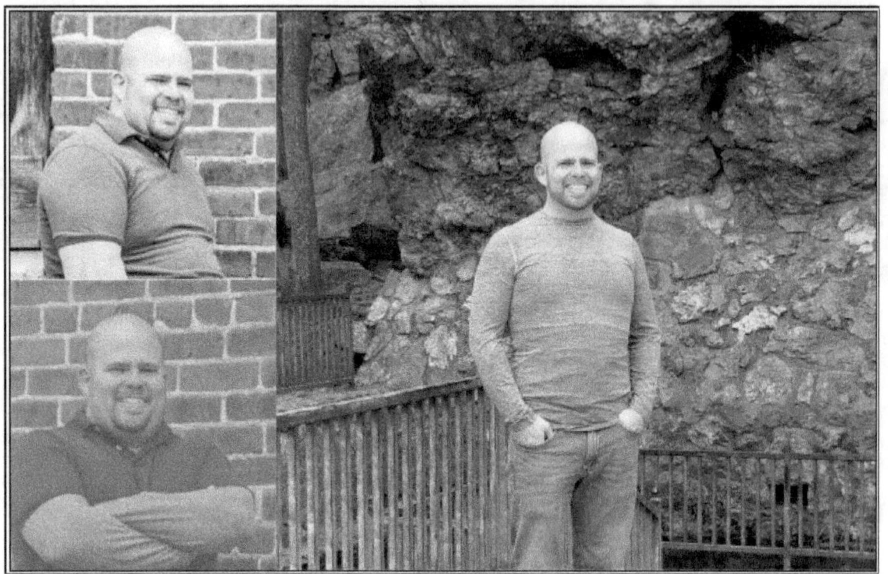

www.ingramcontent.com/pod-product-compliance
Lightning Source LLC
Chambersburg PA
CBHW071215240726

48654CB00009B/799